THE SICK HORSE
Causes, Symptoms, and Treatment

THE SICK HORSE

Causes, Symptoms, and Treatment

Dr. James R. Rooney

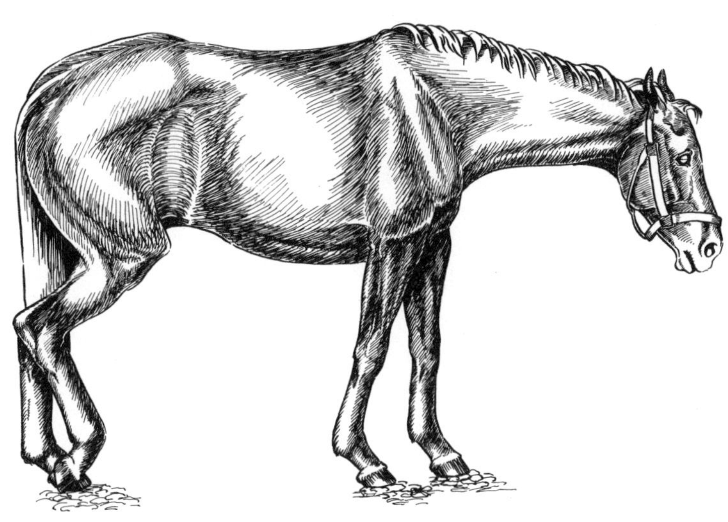

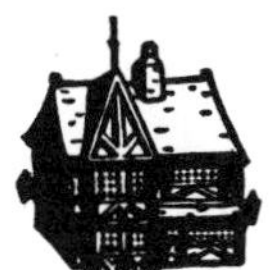

SOUTH BRUNSWICK AND NEW YORK: A. S. BARNES AND COMPANY
LONDON: THOMAS YOSELOFF LTD

A. S. Barnes and Co., Inc.
Cranbury, New Jersey 08512

Thomas Yoseloff Ltd
Magdalen House
136-148 Tooley Street
London SE1 2TT, England

Library of Congress Cataloging in Publication Data

Rooney, James R
The sick horse.

1. Horses—Diseases.   I. Title.
SF951.R686   636.1′08′96   75-22565
ISBN 0-498-01827-X

This book is dedicated
to
Jack Anderson, master Farrier, gentleman

CONTENTS

PREFACE

This book is a companion volume to *The Lame Horse*. In that book, the problems of lameness in horses were considered, primarily in relationship to cause and prevention. In this volume, I shall take up a number of diseases and problems of the modern horse other than lameness. It is my central thesis that broader and deeper understanding of the horse and his problems will enable the horseman to be a more sympathetic and helpful partner with the veterinarian in the prevention and management of the many disease problems which afflict the horse. The informed horseman will demand a higher standard of professional service from his veterinarian, and that is good for both horseman and veterinarian. If you are satisfied with little, that may well be all that you will get. If you want the very best, however, your veterinarian may well be inspired and encouraged to do his best, and that's all to the good of the horse, and that's what this book is all about.

You will not find here a handy guide to clinical signs and do-it-yourself diagnosis and treatment. "My horse has a fever, a runny nose, and holds his tail to the right, so he has right-tail-runny-nose-fever-disease, and the book says that I give him ground wooly caterpillars in two ounces of bourbon." That sort of do-it-yourselfism does not work, and it is both foolish and dangerous to think that it does.

Many of the clinical signs of illness in the horse are quite nonspecific and only indicate that something is wrong and not precisely what is wrong. The trained veterinarian collects all the available signs in a given case, including laboratory tests when indicated. Then, in the light of his knowledge of anatomy, physiology, biochemistry, pathology, etc., he tries to correlate and interpret those signs in order to arrive at a reasonable determination of what problem is present, what organs are involved, how the disease is progressing, what the outcome may be, and, last of all, how to treat it.

Frequently, even the most skillful and experienced veterinarian (or physician, for that matter) cannot determine exactly what is wrong with a given patient. On the basis of experience and training, however, he may be able to come up with a treatment regimen appropriate to the case. Are you laughing? Am I saying that the veterinarian guesses right now and then? Yes, exactly, and with training and experience he guesses right more often than he guesses wrong, and, on the really good days, there's no guessing at all!

A singularly important aspect of dealing with the sick animal is knowing when *not* to do something. At best, medicine acts as an aid to the natural defence mechanisms, helping the animal to affect its own recovery. We do not cure. We help in the cure and should never do things simply for the sake of doing them, running the very real risk of doing more harm than good.

The usual procedure when dealing with the sick animal is to collect the clinical signs, interpret those signs, arrive at a diagnosis, determine the prognosis, and administer treatment. Most of those are obvious, except, perhaps, for prognosis. Let's take a moment to consider that more carefully. It is the one aspect of the veterinarian's work which is least appreciated or understood by the horseman. Prognosis is the process of predicting what the final outcome of the disease, in the given case, will probably be. The prognosis is not often hard fact but, rather, an opinion synthesized from the signs present, the veterinarian's past experience, and that of other veterinarians with similar cases, as well as the treatment techniques available.

Occasionally, the veterinarian will have to say that the prognosis is hopeless. There are several reasons why he may arrive at this conclusion. Humane destruction may be recommended because: 1) The case is truly hopeless. A horse with a broken back and the spinal cord cut in half can never recover. A human in similar straights may live out his life, uncomfortably, in a wheelchair, but that is obviously out of the question for the horse. 2) The disease may be treatable, but the animal has a disease foreign to this country, a disease which should not be allowed to enter and gain a foothold, and the law says that such animals must be destroyed in order to protect the rest of the population. 3) The drugs, surgery, etc. required to affect a cure are beyond the financial means of the horse owner. Often the veterinarian will provide drugs at cost and his own services free in order to save a given animal, but there are, obviously, limits as to how often he can do this and how far he can go. 4) The veterinarian may feel that he must recommend humane destruction because of the certainty that the horseman cannot or will not carry out the tender, loving, nursing care necessary for the animal's recovery. It is true that everyone wants to do everything the first few days, but, as the days and weeks drag by, the duties become onerous, and the recovery is so slow! It may be in the best interests of all concerned to put the animal humanely to sleep in the beginning. 5) In the veterinarian's judgement, the animal will undergo a protracted period of severe pain before recovery can be expected, and this pain is considered to be inhumane. Obviously, this is an area fraught with emotion and difficulty. Often, indeed, it is not the pain experienced by the animal, but the human reaction to that pain which is relevant. 6) The lives of many animals can be saved, but the recovery is incomplete, and the animal is no longer useful for human purposes. A gelding with a broken leg might be saved, but he will never be able to race or jump again.

The physician has a simpler job, in many ways, than the veterinarian. Save life at any cost. The veterinarian must always say: save life, at what cost? And this is cost in terms of money, time, effort, future usefulness, etc. Obviously the veterinarian can be wrong. After a long career of making mistakes, I could hardly deny the possibility! It is important that the case be carefully discussed between the horseman and the veterinarian. In many of the examples given above the prognosis is a function of what the horseman is able and willing to do. With all of the options openly and frankly discussed both the veterinarian and the horseman are in the best position to reach a reasonable conclusion and a mutually agreed-upon prognosis.

On a lighter note, veterinarians of experience have learned to be wary of the owner who says to save the animal "no matter what the cost." That's the owner who never pays the bills. Naturally, he doesn't care what the cost is, since he has no intention of paying anyway!

While what will be said in succeeding pages may be frightening to the reader, the fear is related to the complexity of the problems considered. Only by facing up to complexity and coming to grips with it can we gain understanding. And it is my conviction that, once you understand, the fear will wane, and the horse will be the better for it.

It is clear that we cannot cover every disease entity of the horse in this book. Certain diseases, either foreign to this country or localized in small areas, receive scant or no attention. The aim is to present broad concepts illustrated by specific diseases, and, if you find that your favorite disease has been overlooked, I hope you will be forgiving!

THE SICK HORSE
Causes, Symptoms, and Treatment

1

BREEDING AND BREEDING PROBLEMS

And in the beginning . . . and that's where it all begins. The mare is seasonally polyestrus. That means that she is receptive to the stallion for breeding only at a certain season of the year and only for a certain number of times during that season. In the temperate zones the mare begins to show signs of estrus toward the end of the winter and the beginning of the spring (March, April) and is in full breeding condition during the warm months of May through August (on average).

ESTRUS IN THE MARE

What is an estrous cycle? The full story is very complicated, and can only be discussed in general terms. During the winter months, there is very little activity in the mare's ovary. The pituitary gland, just beneath the brain, is not producing sex hormones, and these hormones are necessary for the activation of the ovary. Without such pituitary stimulus for ovarian activity, the mare does not have estrous cycles. With the coming of spring, the hours of daylight increase. This increase in the amount and duration of light seems to be the most important single factor which stimulates the pituitary to produce the hormones which, in turn, activate the ovary. The first of these pituitary hormones is called follicle stimulating hormone (FSH, for short). FSH travels in the bloodstream from the pituitary to the ovary and, in some way unknown, stimulates the development of the primitive egg cells or ova (ovum = one egg; ova = more than one egg) present in the ovary. The FSH causes these primitive cells to grow and mature and, at the same time, induces the formation of a mantle of cells around the ovum. These "mantle cells" produce fluid and, eventually, the ovum is lying inside a fluid-filled sac. The entire complex, ovum, fluid and mantle cells, is called a Graafian follicle. The fluid contains a hormone, estrogen, produced by the mantle cells. The estrogen escapes from the follicle and circulates in the bloodstream, at first in rather small amounts. Estrogen stimulates the development of the uterus and the mammary gland. As the follicle enlarges, the amount of circulating estrogen increases, and the ovum is maturing and approaching the time for ovulation. The estrogen exerts psychic effects on the mare and, in effect, tells her that it is time for breeding. Simultaneously, the increasing blood levels of estrogen stop the production of FSH by the pituitary, so that no additional primitive ova are stimulated to develop. The estrogen, then, has prepared the uterus, the mammary gland, and the mare's psyche for breeding as the ovum has been developing and preparing itself for fertilization.

When the ovum is ready, the mare will accept the stallion's advances. The estrous cycle reaches its culmination as the ovum bursts from the ovary under the influence of a second pituitary hormone, the luteinizing hormone (LH). The stallion breeds the mare, depositing sperm in her reproductive tract. When the sperm, one of them, reaches and joins the egg, conception has occurred, and a new foal is on the way.

From the practical viewpoint the mare's receptivity to the stallion is all important. How does she let the stallion know that she is ready to be bred? (He's always ready; just waiting for the word!) The question is not an easy one to answer, for the mare's signs to the stallion are in horse language, a language that no human can read completely. One of the obvious signs is "winking." When the stallion approaches the mare, she raises her tail and moves the vestibule (the outer, visible part of the vagina) very rapidly, opening and closing, so that the clitoris which lies just inside the lower part of the vestibule pops in and out. At the same time the mare may squirt small sprays of urine.

If the mare is not in heat, not ready for breeding, she will lay down her ears and indicate very clearly to the stallion that he is not wanted. The absence of this "rejection behavior," then, is a sign to the stallion that his time has come. The mare is quite unique in that the physiological and hormonal changes going on in her body are not tightly tied to the overt or psychological manifestations of heat. That is, the mare's body may be ready for breeding, but she will show no external signs of this fact. Conversely, she may show psychic signs of heat when the physiological mechanisms are not ready. The females of some species show clear physical signs of heat even when no male is about. The mare, however, shows only to the horse. Recognizing this, horsemen have developed the technique of *teasing* as a necessary adjunct to controlled or hand breeding. Under natural conditions, of course, the mare can easily communicate her readiness to the stallion. If mares are not running free with the horse, however, some means must be used to detect the mare in heat, so that she can be taken to the horse. Generally, a vigorous male or even a gelding is used as the teaser. He may be led through the field while the mares are carefully observed for signs of interest in his presence. Alternatively, he may be taken through the barn, pausing at each stall as the handler observes the mare's reactions. The third commonly employed technique is bringing both mare and teaser to a "teasing bar," a sturdy wood panel (part of a fence is often planked in to serve) which keeps the teaser and the mare apart while her reactions to him are observed. The bar may be padded to avoid damage from kicking or bumping. The experienced handler, with a good teaser, can not only detect mares fully in heat but can often form a judgement about mares that are just beginning to come into heat. While the veterinarian can tell a great deal by vaginal examination and palpation of the ovaries, the teaser and his handler know best and are one of a horse farm's best investments.

BREEDING

Under natural breeding conditions the stallion will court the mare for a variable period, nickering, rubbing, grunting and nipping. The length of the courtship will vary from one horse to another. Hand breeding, on the other hand, is completely unnatural. The mare is hobbled to prevent kicking, the tail bandaged, and her entire rear end washed with soap and water. The stallion's penis, too, is thoroughly scrubbed before he is allowed to mount and, often, after the cover has been completed. The mare may be twitched and a heavy canvas or leather cover put over her withers for the stallion that may grip or bite with his teeth while covering. Usually, a breeding roll, 4-6 inches in diameter, is inserted between the mare's rump and the stallion's belly, just above the penis, to prevent too deep a penetration of the penis into the vagina. Such penetration is said to damage the mare's vagina or cervix, though one must wonder what happened to all the wild mares over the centuries!

The horse, under natural or hand breeding conditions, may mount and dismount several times before ejaculating. He may even insert the penis into the vagina but dismount before ejaculation occurs. When ejaculation does occur, the stallion's tail will move up and down rhythmically. This is known as flagging.

The stallion's job is finished, and the millions of sperm which he has placed in the mare now have their big chance! Directed by unknown, but powerful, forces the sperm swim through the uterus and into the oviduct, down which the ovum is making its way to meet them. The strongest and fastest sperm penetrates the ovum and fertilization has been accomplished. Once that first sperm has penetrated the egg, no other sperm may enter. The door is slammed shut. The sperm and ovum blend and the new, combined cell divides rapidly into a cluster of cells as it moves down the oviduct toward the uterus.

Meanwhile, back in the ovary, the Graafian follicle, freed of its ovum, is undergoing interesting and important changes. When rupture (ovulation) of the follicle occurred, releasing the ovum and its surrounding fluid, the resulting space was quickly filled with blood (and is now called a corpus hemorrhagicum: a body of blood, literally). The mantle cells quickly begin to grow into and replace the blood clot. As these cells fill the space formerly occupied by the ovum and its fluid, they produce a hormone, progesterone, which serves to maintain the uterus and its lining in a proper state for the nourishment and maintenance of the embryo, that mass of rapidly dividing cells on its way down the oviduct. Since these hormone-produce cells have a yellowish color, the mass they form in the ovary is called the corpus luteum (body of yellow color).

The corpus luteum forms automatically whether the ovum is fertilized or not. If fertilization does not occur, the corpus luteum will gradually regress and disappear, and the uterus, prepared by the progesterone to receive an embryo, will be "disappointed" and return to its former, resting state. About twenty-one days later, FSH from the pituitary will once again have directed the development of another Graafian follicle, and the estrous cycle repeats itself once again.

INFERTILITY

Before continuing with the story of the fertilized ovum, there are some things to consider that can go wrong with this beautifully organized and controlled system. Why doesn't the mare get in foal? There are three major factors involved: management, the stallion, and the mare.

Management

It has long been traditional that purebred horses have their birthday on the first day of January following their actual birth day. A foal born on January 1st, 1973, then, would actually be a year old on January 1st, 1974. The foal born March 10th, however, is also considered to be one year old on January 1st, 1974, even though he will not be a full year old until March 10th, 1974. As a result, commercial breeders, in particular, try to have mares bred as soon after January 1st as possible, so that the foal will be as old as possible (big and saleable) when January rolls around again. During the short, cold days of January, February, and March, however, many mares simply do not have normal estrous cycles. They either have none at all, irregular ones, or they come into heat and stay in for weeks at a time. For reasons not yet completely understood, the intricately balanced pituitary-ovary system simply does not coordinate well until the days become longer and the weather settled and warm.

Research has clearly shown that the amount of daylight is a major factor. If mares are subjected to artificial daylight during the winter months, they will, on the average, fall into a regular, normal heat pattern earlier than mares subject only to the whim of natural light. It is clear enough, on the other hand, that light is not the only factor. While it may be most important, it does not work alone. It is certainly possible that the experimenters found light easier to work with than other factors and put most of their effort into light since they could work with it. This is hardly a rare phenomenon in scientific research!

As an example of some of those other factors, a few years ago areas in the western part of the United States experienced the worst recorded spring and summer drought in 150 years. Many mares did not show estrous cycles at all while others came in heat in February and stayed in heat through July, but never conceived. It was one of the worst seasons for settling mares that managers and veterinarians in the area could remember. Such events are most obvious in areas subject to large weather and climatic variations from year to year. In other areas, Kentucky, Ohio, and Pennsylvania, for example, such wide swings in the weather from year to year are less common. There are, however, differences from year to year which are subtler and, therefore, may exert more subtle effects, particularly in mares whose reproductive systems are not as secure and well-balanced as one would wish. One thinks of the maiden and old mares specifically.

What is the reason for the mare's seasonal breeding characteristics? If a mare conceives in June, for example she will foal, on average, in May of the next year when the weather is warm and settled, and the new spring grass is present. In other words, seasonal breeding provides for new foals to arrive at the best possible time of year both for weather and food. If there is a terrible drought this year, the grass will still be set back next year, and nature's feedback system simply shuts off breeding, so that there will be no foals to starve to death next spring. Obviously, that story is oversimplified, but the result is the same even if we complicate it considerably. The mare, too, trying to survive the drought conditions, will have a better chance of survival, living to breed another year, if she does not have to feed herself and a fetus when times are hard.

A second major cause of poor conception rates resulting in infertility is the practice of hand breeding. Man determines the match-up between mare and stallion. The mare is hobbled, tail-bandaged, washed and twitched, and the stallion brought in for washing and even manual introduction of the penis into the vagina. Quite apart from the aesthetic abomination involved, the mare is bred once, once only, for that entire heat period. Perhaps, if the stallion is available (and that is man's planning as well), she may be bred back once more during that heat period. Twice, that's all. From numerous observations it is clear that, in the natural state, the stallion will cover the mare a number of times during the course of a single heat. (Though somewhat extreme, one young stud was observed to cover a filly twenty-three times during a three day heat period, and that was only during the day!)

While perhaps of lesser importance in the overall picture, individual mare peculiarities certainly do operate. I have, on a number of occasions, seen mares, hobbled and twitched though they were, absolutely refuse to permit a certain stallion to cover them. A second stallion is brought in, and the breeding is quickly done without the mare batting an eyelash. The mare need never have seen either stallion previously. It is probably true that the stallion will cover anything that will stand still long enough, including an artificial vagina, but mares can be most selective.

Infertility of the Stallion

Infertility of the stallion, the inability to deliver sufficient numbers of vigorous sperm for the fertilization of the egg, is a major factor in modern horse breeding practise.

One of the more common, recognized, causes of poor stallion performance is the psychological factor. The young stallion, new to the breeding ranks, must be handled with great care. While some young males know immediately what is expected and get on with the job, others are not at all sure what to do or how to do it. In the wild state, the young male learns from the example of his elders and is helped along by the proximity, during the breeding season, of the number of mares in heat. Under hand breeding conditions, however, the young male, whose closest associations for several years have been with man rather than other horses, may have his problems. The young stallion's first mare should be quiet and receptive. She can, in effect, train the horse and encourage him. (There are some human societies with this same interesting concept.) While difficult to prove, experience indicates that poor or reluctant breeding performance in later years can often be traced back to psychological trauma during the stallion's first breeding season (if not, indeed, to his first mare).

The young stallion must be treated gently and carefully by his human handler. The handler must be patient, allowing the stallion time to talk to the mare, move around, and gradually fill in for himself what he is supposed to do. Such patience may be rewarded the first time. If not, the stallion may be brought back to the mare later in the day, until, gradually, his courage increases (a major factor), and he is ready to try. Failing this, it may be necessary to turn the horse out in a paddock next to the mare until he is ready. Above all, one must be patient! The human handler can inflict as much psychological trauma as the unwilling mare.

A singular cause of breeding inefficiency is simply lack of a regular routine. The stallion does not get enough daily exercise and becomes fat and indolent. He should be fed on a regular basis, exercised on a regular basis, and always handled by the same person, if possible. Some stallions are said to perform better if they are kept away from other horses, but most seem to require at least the regular sight and sound of others of their own kind.

Masturbation is said to be a major factor in poor breeding performance and relative infertility. The semen count (number of normal sperm in an ejaculate) may decline, and the stallion lose libido as a result of masturbation. The horseman may not be aware of this problem since masturbation is, as a rule, a solitary vice. While the experience of years certainly supports the idea that masturbation can be a problem in lowering fertility, one must wonder how much of this experience has been colored by the Victorian horror of the practise in the human (attributing to it everything from insanity to boils). There are, if one believes or can prove that it is a problem, devices to prevent or, at least, inhibit the horse from indulging. Such devices are not innocuous, however, and should only be used with the advice of the veterinarian or an experienced stallion handler. Masturbation, like most vices in horses, is the direct result of boredom, inactivity, and unnatural isolation of the animal from others of his own kind. One must remember that the horse is a most gregarious, social animal.

Overbreeding, too frequent use of the stallion, may lead to a decline in semen quality and poor conception rates during the latter part of the breeding season. Also, the stallion may simply become fatigued or lose interest; too much of a good thing, one might say.

Nutrition is frequently blamed for infertility when no other explanation is readily available. It is certainly true that the stallion in poor condition, whether it be from illness or an inadequate type or amount of food, will have lowered fertility to the point of complete sterility. A more common problem, already alluded to, is obesity, too much nutrition either from overfeeding, lack of exercise or both. While obesity may not lower the sperm count, it does reduce libido.

Infection of the stallion's genitalia (reproductive organs) is an occasional problem. *Coital exanthema* is a virus disease which causes multiple blisters, pustules, and ulcers on the penis. The virus is readily transmitted to mares during breeding. The stallion may refuse to breed because of pain and should not be bred in any case in order to avoid transmitting the disease to the mares. The disease is self-limiting and without untoward after-effects, but it can seriously disrupt the breeding season.

Bacterial infections of one type or another may localize in the testes or one of the other sex organs. In the former case fertility is sharply and usually permanently decreased if not completely lost. In the case of localization of infection in the prostate or seminal vesicles, the stallion may remain at least partially fertile but can transmit the infection to susceptible mares. Treatment, in either case, is difficult, not often completely successful, and must be under professional supervision.

An important consideration in partial or complete infertility of the male is genetic factors. Examination of the ejaculate of a genetically infertile stallion will reveal few or no normal, living sperm cells. Microscopic examination of the testes shows that the normal processes of sperm formation are not proceeding, but there will be no indication why they are not. It does seem clear that, in the long run, man is at fault. Let us assume that there is a partially infertile stallion in a herd of wild horses. He is partially infertile because of the random mutation of a gene. The stallion has adequate libido and breeds his mares dutifully. Few of them get in foal, however. Any male offspring (and perhaps female as well) will, like their father, be partially or completely infertile. With few progeny and these few afflicted, that stallion's line will quickly die out. Infertility, under natural conditions, is distinctly self-limiting, in other words.

Man, however, does not select stallions for fertility alone. He selects for appearance, racing speed, jumping, whatever. If a partially infertile stallion was a champion but gets only half of his mares in foal, he is doing better than the fully fertile nonchampion, in man's terms. There are few offspring, but they are winners! Only complete sterility will wipe itself out when man is the primary agent of genetic selection.

Mares may, of course, participate in this same genetic process. If a great stakes mare produces only three foals in her lifetime, but one of them is a stakes winner, the owner may consider his investment worthwhile. But, that stakes winning offspring will perpetuate the mare's relative infertility! No Hereford bull or cow could get away with it. The bull, and cow, must produce numbers as well as quality. The stallion or mare need only produce quality, no matter how few the numbers. I remember one great race mare who was bred regularly every year for fifteen years and never got in foal. The veterinarians knew she wouldn't because there was a congenital defect of her reproductive tract: part of the uterus was missing. Sperm deposited in the vagina had no way to reach the egg in the oviduct.

Hormones are often suggested as a cause of infertility in both stallions and mares, but there is little hard evidence to support the contention either in the stallion or the mare. In recent years, there seems to have been an upsurge of cases of immature, incompletely formed sperm appearing in the ejaculates of stallions just entering the breeding ranks after a racing career. Simply put, this means the sperm are leaving the testes earlier than they should, before they are mature and capable of fertilizing the ovum. The reason for this is not clear, at this time, but researchers suspect that some of the many drugs administered to horses in training may be responsible. Further work may clarify that, but one must always be suspicious of the genetic factor!

Infertility of the Mare

Turning now to the mare one finds a great deal more information available on the causes and nature of infertility. (I wonder if the new wave of female veterinarians, with a different viewpoint, may not do as well by the stallion?) The most common and important cause of infertility of the mare is infection of the uterus by bacterial organisms. A mare with such an infection typically comes into heat and has a dirty, thin, watery exudate seeping from the vulva. Despite repeated breeding she does not get in foal. When the veterinarian examines her with a speculum, he sees a reddened, inflamed lining of the vagina and cervix. There may be a frothy, dirty, grey exudate sticking to the walls and sloshing about on the floor of the vagina. These signs of infection of the vagina and cervix are invariably accompanied by infection of the uterus as well. The technical terms which you will hear are vaginitis (inflammation of the vagina), cervicitis (inflammation of the cervix), and endometritis (endo means lining, metri means uterus and itis means inflammation (inflammation of the lining of the uterus).

The veterinarian may take a sample of the exudate for culture. The sample is placed on plates of agar containing substances which will allow and encourage bacteria to grow. Examination of the agar plates once the bacteria have grown will allow the veterinarian or the laboratory to identify what type or types of bacteria are causing the infection. From previous research and experience, the veterinarian will know which antibiotic or combination of antibiotics to place in the uterus in order to eliminate the infection. There are also laboratory tests, called antibiotic sensitivity tests, which can help in deciding which antibiotic to use. The veterinarian may also make use of the relatively new technique of biopsy of the uterine lining. That is, he will take a small piece of tissue from the uterus for culture and for examination under the microscope. The full value of this technique is still being determined. The rationale for its use is that if the tissue is normal apart from the acute infection, the prognosis for the future breeding life of the mare is quite good. If, on the other hand, there is significant, permanent, chronic damage to the lining of the uterus, the prognosis is not nearly as favorable. The antibiotics can eliminate the bacteria causing the acute infection, but the lining of the uterus is so badly damaged that there is little hope that it can maintain pregnancy.

For many years infection in any part of the body has been thought of in rather simplistic terms. Bacteria and the products of their living, eating and dying are foreign to the animal. Materials which are foreign incite the body or a part of the body (in this case the uterus) to mount a defensive reaction against them, and this defensive reaction is inflammation. Inflammation consists of the following cardinal signs: redness, heat, swelling, pain and loss of use. Virtually all of these signs are the result of increased blood flow to the affected area, and that increased flow is in response to the presence of foreign materials and the damage done to the tissues by those foreign materials. Microscopically, one can see white blood cells moving out of the blood stream into the area in order to engulf and destroy the invaders.

It is clear that the greatest majority of bacteria (as well as fungi) which enter the uterus are quickly and immediately destroyed by the inflammatory reaction. If one pours streptococci (one of the commonest bugs infecting the mare's uterus) into the uterus of a normal mare, for example, there is a quick and violent inflammatory reaction, and the infection is soon disposed of. In some mares, however, the infection is not eliminated but persists and perks along slowly. There is inflammation, but it is less than maximal, and the infecting organisms are not destroyed. These mares do not get in foal because the lining of the infected uterus is being damaged by the bacteria and is in no condition to allow the survival and growth of a fertilized embryo.

The questions to be answered, then, are: 1) How do the bacteria get into the uterus, and 2) why do they call forth a maximal inflammatory reaction in some mares and not in others?

1) All common bacterial infections of the uterus enter by way of the vulva, through the vagina and cervix, and into the uterus. Any time, then, that the vulva is open, bacteria can enter. The vulva is open (or readily openable) during estrus. During estrus, however, the hormone, estrogen, renders the reproductive tract resistant to bacterial infection. It

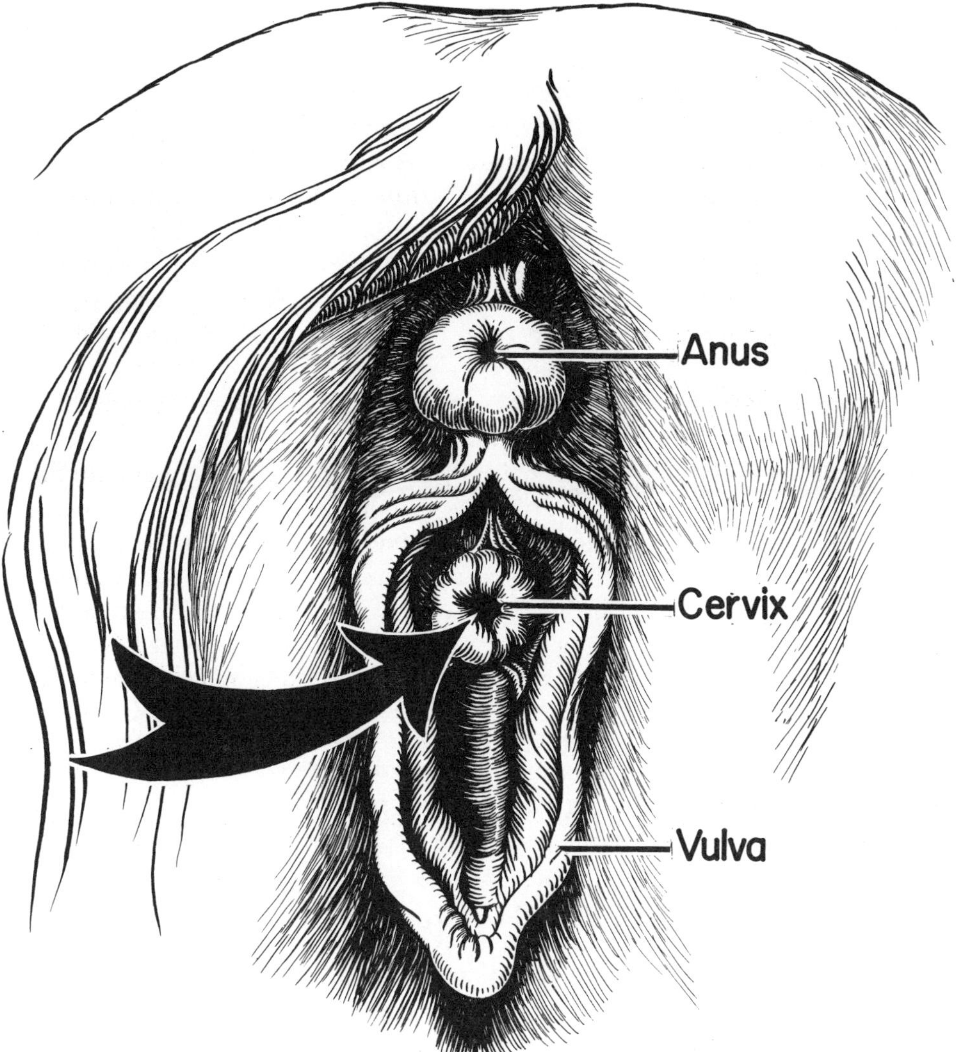

Fig. 1   Schematic interpretation of a wind-sucking mare. The lips of the vulva are open, and the mare is aspirating air into the vagina, cervix and uterus.

became apparent years ago that certain mares, prone to this type of low-grade, persisting infection were what are called "wind-suckers." That is, they, for some reason, open the lips of the vulva and aspirate air into the vagina. Since bacteria, and particularly streptococci, are always around horses, they could enter the vagina with this aspirated air. Other mares had loose or atonic (lacking in normal tightness or tone) vulvae which allowed air to enter with or without wind-sucking. A third category of mares had tipped vulvae, the upper end being farther forward than the

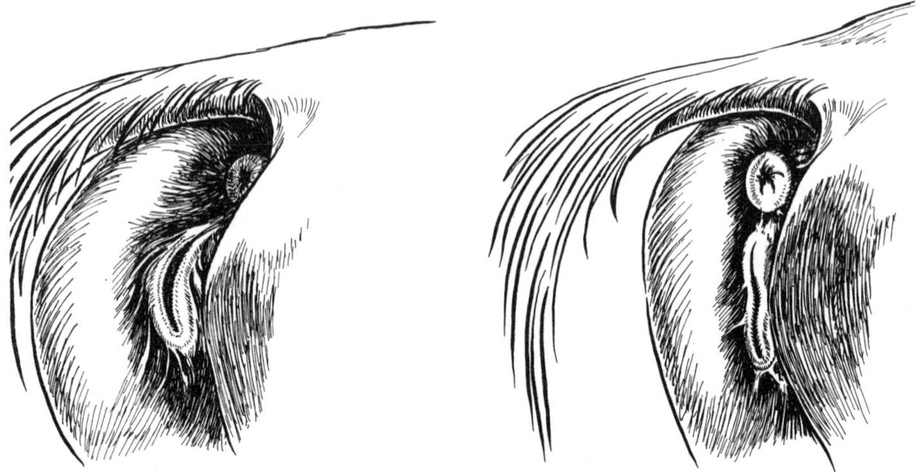

Fig. 2 Normal, vertical orientation of the anus (above) and vulvar lips to the right. The "tipped" vulva is to the left.

lower end. This is a particularly bad conformation. Whenever a mare defecates, some fluid can run down from the anus on to the vulva. If the vulva is straight up and down and of normal tone, the fecal water will simply run off. If the vulva is tipped forward, however, the fluid may run into the vagina, introducing bacteria and infection.

Many years ago, two pioneering horse veterinarians, Drs. Dimock and Caslick, recognized this problem and developed the operation still known as the Caslick operation. They sutured the upper two-thirds (approximately) of the vulva closed. While this allowed the urine to be voided, it reduced or prevented wind-sucking, tightened the atonic vulva, and shut off the entrance for fecal fluid.

While the Caslick operation has helped many mares to get in foal, it is not a panacea. The vulvar opening is so small after suturing that breeding and foaling are impossible. Before either event, then, it is necessary to have the veterinarian reopen the vulva and close it again later.

There is no explanation for the mare with a normal vulva who sucks air except to say that it is a vice, some sort of psychological quirk. Atonic and tipped vulvae, however, can be partially explained. The tipped vulva may be hereditary. The mare is born that way, and her daughters are very apt to be the same way. Apart from that, the vulva will tend to tip farther forward as the mare ages. This is the result of several factors, primarily repeated pregnancies with gradual loss of tone in the reproductive tissues (old age "wear and tear"). Instead of involuting tightly after foaling the uterus may remain large and baggy, hanging down in the abdominal cavity, thereby pulling the vulva into the tipped-forward position. Often, accompanying this age-related loss of tone, urine will tend to pool on the floor of the vagina. In this case, the loss of tone involves the vaginal muscle and, perhaps, the urinary bladder muscle as well.

The atonic vulva is seen most frequently in older mares and must be related to wear and tear, the inevitable ravages of age. Repeated Caslick operations, too, will contribute to loss of tone. Both the tipped and atonic vulva are seen in young mares in poor condition as the result of inadequate nutrition and/or debilitating illness.

2) Even with the Caslick operation, however, there are many mares that can develop low-grade, persisting infections. They seem unable to mount an inflammatory reaction of sufficient magnitude to throw off the infection. Why? We don't know, and that's the truth. Here is what we do know. When the mare is in the estrogen phase of her cycle, in heat, the uterus and vagina are resistant to bacterial invasion. This is reasonable. Since the cervix is wide open, and the stallion will be entering the mare, bacteria will, inevitably, be introduced, and estrogen provides protection against these bacterial invaders. No one knows how estrogen exerts this effect, only that it does. Once the heat period is over, and the progesterone produced by the corpus luteum takes over, the uterus is much more easily infected. Again, this is reasonable. The progesterone conditions the uterus to receive, support, and nourish the embryo, and when in this state, the uterus can do the same for bacteria. Normally, the cervix will be tightly closed once progesterone has taken over, however, and the bacteria cannot gain entrance to the uterus. Obviously, there is the potential in such a complicated system for slight mistiming in the shift from one hormone to the other, the timely closing of the cervix, inadequate amounts of estrogen, or some form of blockage of the estrogen antibacterial effect. Although there is such a potential, we have no evidence that any of these things actually do happen. In fact, the defect in the easily infected mare may be related to some factor or factors other than hormonal, such as inadequate amount or type of antibody production. Rather than continue to waffle on about this, I repeat: we don't know and that's the truth. Only research can provide an answer.

Hormonal disturbances are a well-known cause of infertility among females of a number of species. The situation is unclear and incompletely understood in the mare. It is clear, though, that the failure of mares to cycle regularly and conceive early in the year, during the winter months, is related to uneven, unsynchronized hormonal activity. As we have already discussed, light stimulates the pituitary to produce the master hormones, FSH and LH, which control the ovary. The fluctuations of light during the winter and, probably, fluctuation in the "start-up" process in the pituitary itself, can lead to a shallow estrus (incompletely expressed external signs), no estrus (known as anestrus), or widely fluctuating signs of estrus. There is no reasonable treatment for this other than waiting for spring. If the abnormal heat periods continue into the spring, there is the temptation to initiate hormone therapy. From what I can gather, the results of administering hormones to mares have been, at best, inconsistent, uncontrolled, and useless. Regular teasing, time and prayer seem to be the treatments of choice. Regular teasing, in particular, provides regular stimulation to the psyche and endocrine system of the mare and seems to help the process of settling down and establishing normal rhythmns.

Nymphomania does occur in mares. Some nymphomaniacal mares ovulate normally and get in foal without difficulty, though willing to accept the stallion at almost any time. Other mares may show almost continuous signs of estrus although the ovaries are completely inactive. Any given mare with such signs may or may not be willing to accept the stallion even though she shows all the overt signs of estrus. Irritation of the clitoris by some foreign material such as weed seeds, hairs, or plant fibers, may be the cause in a few cases. More often, the cause cannot be discovered, and we must fall back upon "psychological factors" which are not understood. In a number of species cystic ovaries accompany nymphomania, but this is not true in the mare. Fortunately nymphomania is uncommon since, with the exception of clitoris irritation, there is nothing we can do about it.

Commonly fillies just off the racetrack have difficulty getting in foal. While either nervousness, poor condition, or sexual immaturity may be the problem, often the cause is the heat-suppressing, male-type hormones the filly has received while at the track. The suppressive effects of these hormones may persist directly or indirectly for a considerable period of time. Time and tender, loving care are indicated. Eventually, barring other problems, the filly's endocrine system will rebalance itself, and conception will become possible.

Even without the suppressive effects of male hormones, the successful race mare may present difficulties as a broodmare. While objective proof is not available, I might suggest that the best race mares have a more masculine turn of mind and body. Males, as a rule, make better racing individuals than females, and those mares which more closely rival the males may be biased psychologically and hormonally toward the male constitution. An adjunct to this concept is the observation that mares tend to go sour on racing earlier than males. This "sourness" often appears during the four year old year when the filly is reaching sexual maturity and the biological drive becomes more important than the training of man.

Several points remain. Mares may fail to show signs of estrus for any one of several reasons. First, and obviously, the mare may be pregnant! It is not invariable that a pregnant mare will not show signs of heat. Some do and some do not.

Some mares will cycle normally, developing follicles and ovulating and yet never showing overt, physical signs of heat. The cause is unknown but probably related to unknown psychological factors. In the same category may be the mare who does show appropriate signs of estrus and ovarian activity but simply does not get in foal to a particular stallion, though able to get in foal to another stallion. There may be psychological factors here or, perhaps a matching of genes between the two which is lethal to the embryo in the very first stages of development.

The corpus luteum may be retained in the ovary, producing progesterone, for a considerable period even though there is no foal present in the uterus. The mare, of course, will not come in heat as long as progesterone is being produced. Eventually, this corpus luteum will regress, and normal cycling will resume. The cause of this retention of the corpus luteum is unknown. Spurious pregnancy (the mare is bred and does not come in heat again for several months only to return to normal cycling without evidence of abortion) may be an example of retention of the corpus luteum. It is not always easy to diagnose this problem since the corpus luteum is usually deeply buried in the ovary, and, therefore, not palpable (felt through the rectum) by the veterinarian.

A known cause of retention of the corpus luteum is the presence of severe infection and damage to the lining (the endometrium) of the uterus. The disappearance or regression of the corpus luteum is caused by a factor or factors produced by the endometrium. If a foal is present or if the lining has been heavily damaged by infection, this factor may not be produced and the corpus luteum persists.

Lactation and nursing, also, will suppress ovulation in some mares. The mechanism is not understood and, for the time being, one can only wait until the foal is weaned even if this means that the mare only has a foal every other year.

DEVELOPMENT OF THE FERTILIZED EGG

Rapid cell division begins soon after the sperm has entered the egg. Before fertilization, both egg and sperm each had only one half of the appropriate, normal number of chromosomes. The fertilized egg has a full set, one half from the male and one half from the female. The fertilized egg divides into two new cells, then four, then eight, and so on. Quickly, this new mass of cells begins to differentiate into the several cell and tissue types which will eventually form the skin, bone, nervous tissue, gut, etc. The cell mass is now an embryo. As it is growing, dividing and differentiating, it moves down the oviduct to the uterus. In addition to its own, intrinsic organs and tissues, the embryo begins to form the four membranes or sacs of the placenta which will house and nourish it during the eleven months in the uterus.

The first of these sacs is the yolk sac. It provides a store of nourishment for the embryo during the first days of its existence. This is the same structure as the yolk of the chicken egg, but is smaller and quickly used up by the developing embryo. The chicken embryo feeds on the yolk sac during its entire time within the egg. The horse embryo uses up the yolk

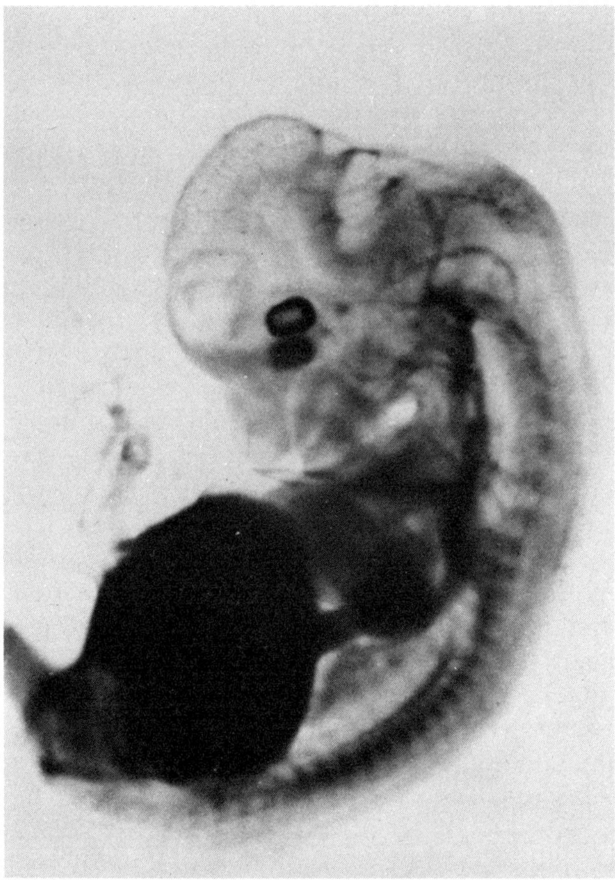

Fig. 3 An early horse fetus. The specimen has been cleared in order to show some of the internal organs. The black eyes, above, and the large, dark mass of the liver, below, are particularly striking.

in a short while and becomes dependent upon nutrients brought to it by other parts of the placenta. The sac immediately around the embryo encloses the amniotic cavity and is known as the amnion. The fluid in this cavity is in direct contact with the embryo. As the embryo grows into a fetus (the change in name is somewhat arbitrary and usually given as 30 days) amniotic fluid is swallowed into the lungs and intestinal tract. There is a continuous flow, apparently, of amniotic fluid into the fetus and out again, the significance of which is not known.

The second cavity, surrounding the amniotic, is the allantoic cavity. The membrane enclosing this cavity, the allantois, is fused with the outermost membrane, the chorion, and ·the two combined, fused membranes are known as the chorioallantois or chorioallantoic membrane. The allantoic cavity is continuous with the urinary bladder of the fetus and apparently serves, at least in part, as a reservoir for the urine which the fetus produces during intrauterine life.

The outer layer, the chorion, serves as the exchange surface with the inner lining of the uterus, the endometrium. The mare's blood flows through the endometrium and the fetal blood through the chroion, and carbon dioxide, oxygen, and nutrients are exchanged between the two circulations. In many other species there is much closer contact between the two circulations (maternal and fetal) than is true of the horse.

During the first 100 days or so of pregnancy the fetal blood exchanges gases and nutrients with the maternal blood through fluid present in the space between endometrium and placenta. This fluid is apparently produced by the uterine glands. Somewhere between 50 and 100 days (the matter is in some dispute) the chorion develops small, tree-like villi or fingerlike projections which fit closely into the glands and folds of the endometrium. The exchange surfaces (villi and endometrium) are now in very close contact, and nutrients and gases can move directly from endometrium to chorion and vice versa.

Until about 100 days the fetus is floating about inside the several membranes with no attachment to the endometrium. With the formation of villi, attachment to the endometrium begins. This process always starts at the junction of the body of the uterus with one or the other of the two horns of the uterus. As the fetus grows, it pushes its placenta in front of it to fill the body of the uterus and the one horn. Eventually the placenta will be pushed into the opposite horn as well. The first horn of the uterus to fill with placenta, and fetus, is called the pregnant horn while the other, reasonably enough, is called the nonpregnant horn. (This description is oversimplified. The placenta grows and is not literally "pushed.")

Meanwhile, back in the ovary, some strange and wonderful things are happening. The first corpus luteum, the one which formed when the follicle ruptured, persists, producing progesterone, for at least 45 days.

Meanwhile, several new follicles are developing. They may or may not ovulate (the evidence is unclear) but, in any case, they form corpora lutea (that's the plural for corpus luteum) which add to progesterone production and gradually take over as the first corpus luteum fades away. The mare may show signs of heat while this "second wave" of follicles is developing. Obviously one does not rush to breed the mare again without ascertaining first whether or not she is in foal!

The second crop of corpora lutea last until roughly 150 days at which time they, too, fade away. After that the progesterone necessary to maintain pregnancy is produced by the placenta itself.

During the first two to three months of pregnancy, the fetus forms all the tissues and organs that it will have at birth. After three months, then, pregnancy is, for the fetus, primarily a matter of growing in size. Other things are happening but the main job is to grow.

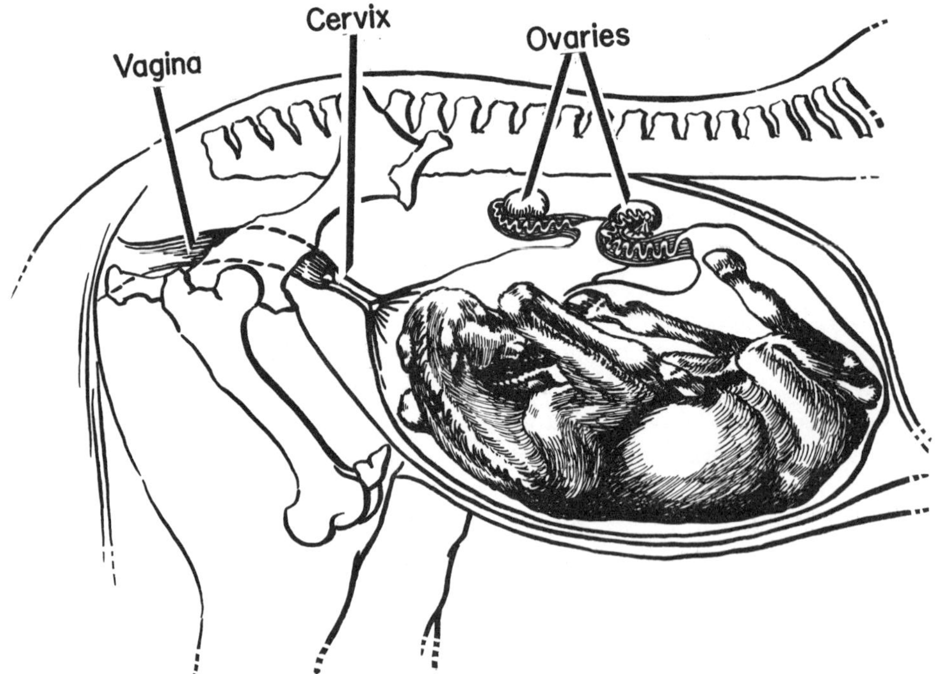

Fig. 4 The well-developed, growing fetus within the uterus.

2
FETAL DEATH AND ABORTION

There are, needless to say, many things that can go wrong during this complicated developmental process. Both external and internal factors can operate to either distort the development of the fetus or stop it altogether.

EARLY ABORTION

Between conception and about 100 days, 5-8% of the embryo-fetuses will be lost. These figures are not quite accurate since they are based on rectal diagnosis between the twentieth and forty-fifth days of pregnancy and again at 90-150 days, but they are reasonably close. The embryo may die in the uterus and be so decomposed and dissolved by the time it is aborted that it cannot be found, or identified if it is found. The few that have been examined during this early period have all had evidence of bacterial infection. It seems reasonable to say that bacteria already present in the uterus or introduced at the time of breeding infected the fetus, causing its death and subsequent abortion. As soon as the fetus dies (or quickly thereafter) the cervix opens in preparation for abortion. Bacteria can enter the uterus once the cervix has opened and infect or infest the already dead fetus. Since the fetus, at this time, cannot mount an inflammatory reaction to the bacteria even if it is alive, we cannot use that as a clue for determining whether the bacteria invaded

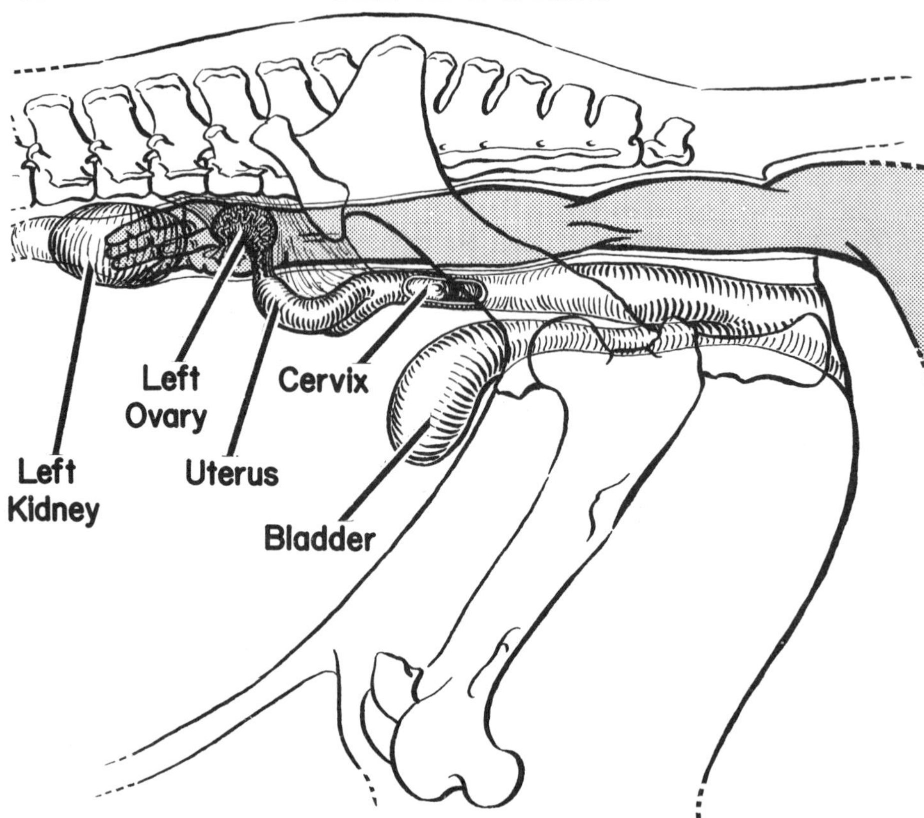

Fig. 5 A schematic drawing of the veterinarian's arm and hand (shaded) in the rectum in order to examine the kidney and reproductive tract.

and killed the fetus or invaded the fetus after it had died for some other reason.

Many of these early abortions may be the result of congenital or genetic defects which are so lethal that the embryo dies very soon after cell multiplication begins. There is recent evidence from biopsy studies of the uterus that severe scarring of the uterus with subsequent loss of normal endometrium for supporting the development of the fetus and its membranes can be a real factor in the cause of these early abortions.

FOUR TO SIX MONTH ABORTION

There are a number of abortions during the 4th to 6th month of pregnancy. The fetuses are markedly decomposed and laboratory procedures do not help to determine why they died and were aborted.

Since this 4-6 month period is the time when the source of progesterone for maintenance of pregnancy is shifting from ovary to placenta, it is possible that there is an error during this shift, or a mistiming of the shift, which causes the abortion. There is, further, evidence that severe stressing of the mare (such as shipping) during this critical shift-over period may add up to abortion. Progesterone has been given by injection to try and overcome this problem, but without marked success, probably because the dosage has been too low and administered at too long intervals.

TWIN ABORTION

Year in and year out, the most important single cause of abortion in light horses is twinning. In any given year, on any given farm, some other cause may predominate, but, overall, twinning is the most important cause of abortion. In many species, twinning is not abnormal though less common than single births (human and cow, for example). In the mare, however, the entire endometrial-chorial interface is necessary for the successful growth and development of one foal. Whenever that total

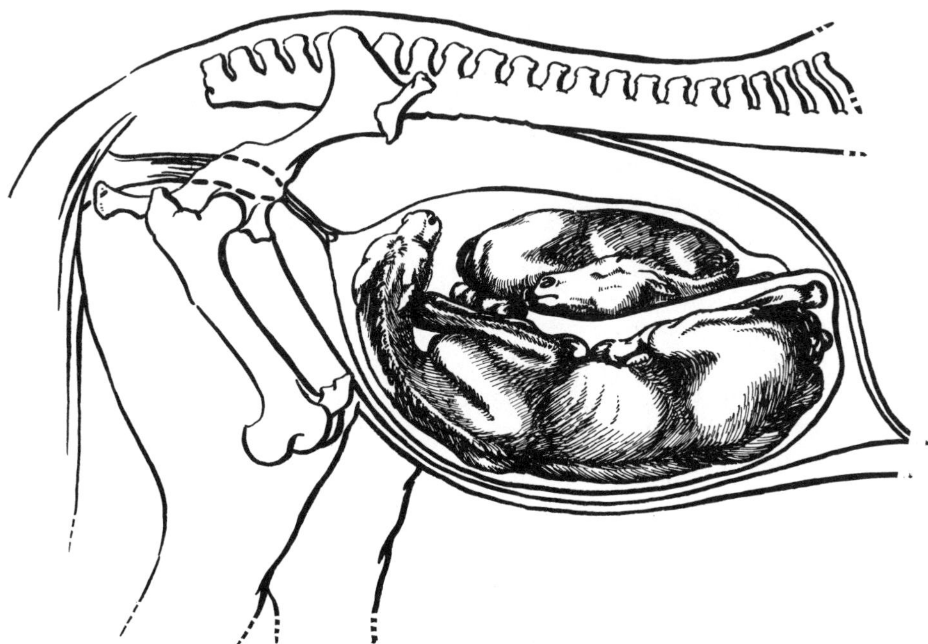

Fig. 6 A twin pregnancy. The larger fetus is below and the smaller which will die first is above.

surface is not available, fetal distress, death, and abortion are to be expected.

Most twins (among Thoroughbreds and Standardbreds at least) are fraternal. That is, the two fetuses come from two separate and distinct eggs which leave the ovary or ovaries at about the same time. The rare identical twin pregnancy (I've only seen one) is the result of splitting of one fertilized egg into two and the subsequent development of two identical fetuses.

The reason for the abortion of a twin pregnancy is quite clear. As already discussed, the villi begin to form on the chorion between 50-100 days. The villi will form, however, only if the chorion is in contact with normal endometrium. Since the two chorions of the twins expand and come into contact with each other before this time, villi cannot form on those chorial surfaces in contact with each other and not, therefore, in contact with endometrium. As a result each twin has less chorial-endometrial exchange surface than it should. Without villi, the exchange surface is much less efficient. As the fetuses increase in size, they compete for the available exchange surface and, inevitably, one gets ahead of the other. It receives more of the nutrients and oxygen, growing faster and larger than its mate. Eventually the smaller twin dies because it can neither acquire enough nutrients to grow nor enough oxygen to stay alive.

The mare, in some way unknown, "senses" that a fetus is dead. She shows signs identical to those of impending foaling. The tissues around the vulva loosen, the udder enlarges ("making bag") and a vaseline-like secretion is forced out of the teats ("waxing"). Milk may run from the udder. These signs may be followed, in a short time, by abortion, or they may disappear only to reappear some time later and be followed by abortion. The dead twin lies inside its membranes and simply dries up and decomposes, while the live fetus continues to grow. Eventually, the live fetus, too, will reach a critical point. It does not have enough exchange surface (villi cannot form now, only at the earlier time) and, reaching a critical size, there will not be sufficient oxygen coming from the placenta. The mare aborts both fetuses, the long-dead one and the newly suffocated one. One fetus is always larger than the other, and the larger is always fresh while the smaller is, of course, rotten. It should be noted that "larger" is a relative term. The fetus is never as big as a single fetus at the same stage of pregnancy.

Twin abortions occur at any time from about six months to term though most occur around 7 to 10 months. Occasionally, a mare will abort one of the twins and retain the other for a short period. Also, she may abort and the small, decomposed fetus be overlooked in the field or bedding. Careful examination of the placental membranes will clearly show that it was a twin abortion even if only one fetus is found.

Why do mares conceive twins if it is abormal? We don't know. Since many mares tend to have twins time and again, it seems probable that the tendency to twinning is hereditary.

Careful rectal palpation by an experienced veterinarian during estrus can be of assistance in avoiding twins. If his hand can detect two follicles developing simultaneously in the ovaries, he may advise not breeding the mare during that heat period. There are no guarantees, however, since a second follicle can be developing deep within the ovary beyond his probing fingers.

An occasional twin pregnancy may go to term with the birth of two live miniature foals. Such an outcome is uncommon and does not, in any way, alter the fact that twin pregnancy is abnormal in the horse.

The question of superovulation comes up periodically. That is, if a mare is bred twice during a single heat period (or even two different heat periods) by the same or different stallions, and a twin pregnancy results, one might think that two different follicles were ovulated at very different times rather than at about the same time. It really is not an important question since the end result is the same, either way. This impression of superovulation is often based on the different size of the two fetuses or foals, but, as we have seen, this is a matter of competition between the two within the uterus and not necessarily the result of conception at widely different times.

PLACENTAL DISEASE

The basic cause of fetal death and abortion in twin pregnancy is inadequate placentation. There is simply not enough endometria-chorial exchange surface to support two fetuses through pregnancy. A similar situation can develop with the single fetus if the placenta is improperly formed or diseased in any one of a variety of ways. No matter what the nature of the placental abnormality, the cause of abortion, in the final analysis, will be starvation and suffocation of the fetus because of inadequate placental exchange surface.

The clinical signs of impending abortion (making bag, waxing) are essentially the same as those preceeding twin abortion.

Hypovillation

The first type of placental abnormality is called hypovillation. Hypo is a prefix meaning too little or too few, while villation refers to the villi of the chorion. Hypovillation, then, is simply too few villi. This is the same problem that occurs with twin pregnancy, except that, in this case, there is only one fetus and no apparent reason for the paucity of villi. As with many placental abnormalities, however, the cause is unknown, although there are two possible reasons. The first is that hypovillation is a congenital defect of the chorion. That is, the villi fail to form because of a disturbance in the early development of the placenta. We are aware of congenital defects of the fetus—cleft palates, contracted limbs, knockknees, undeveloped eyes, etc., but rarely does one think of defects of the placenta itself. Since the placenta and fetus develop from the same fertilized egg, it is not unreasonable that congenital malformations could affect either or both.

A second cause of hypovillation can be disease of the endometrium. That is, if there has been infection of the endometrium with scarring and destruction of the normal architecture, the endometrium may be so changed that it can no longer induce the formation of villi when in contact with the chorion. There is clinical and pathological evidence for such a cause.

Body Pregnancy

This is an example of what I consider to be a congenital malformation of the placenta. It has already been noted that the fetus implants at the junction of the body and one horn of the uterus. With the body pregnancy, however, implantation occurs at the usual site, but the placenta and fetus expand only into the body of the uterus and not into the horns.

Most body pregnancies are aborted during the seventh month of pregnancy. This tells us something most useful and interesting. The placental exchange area provided by the body portion of the placenta alone is sufficient to support and maintain the fetus for about seven months. The additional surface area provided by the pregnant horn, then, is what is necessary for the remaining four months. I do not mean that the body alone carries the fetus for seven months, and then the horn "kicks in" for the next four months. Rather, the surface area represented by the body equals seven months and the surface area of the horn represents four months. In the hypovillated placenta discussed above, then, one can make an estimate of the surface area lacking villi and correlate that with the time of abortion. If the nonvillated area is about five month's worth, the fetus is aborted at about six months. If the area is nine months, abortion is expected at two months. If the area is three months, the fetus is aborted about eight months. In the case of body pregnancy, as noted, abortion is at seven months.

Bacterial and Fungal Infections

A number of abortions in any given year are caused by bacterial infections which gain entrance to the uterine cavity when, and if, the cervix opens. The bacteria can infect the placenta or the fetus or both at the same time. The endometrial-chorial interface is an active site for the exchange of nutrient materials and gases. It is warm, moist, nutrient-rich, admirably suited to maintain the fetus and, as a result, is an ideal culture ground for bacteria as well. When the bacteria enter and begin to multiply, the endometrium and the allantochorion respond to their presence with an inflammatory reaction. The inflammation and its consequences inhibit or stop the proper exchange of nutrients and gases between mare and fetus. If large areas of exchange surface are involved, the fetus suffocates (the same process as with twins and other forms of placental disease).

Bacterial infections usually cause abortion during the 6th to 9th month whether the placenta or the fetus or both are infected. Streptococcus is the common organism, but that is of less importance than the manner of invasion as we shall discuss below.

Fungal infections of the placenta generally cause abortion during the last three months of pregnancy (though the infection probably starts earlier, 6th to 9th month). The fungus (usually an *Aspergillus*) grows on the surface of the chorion in the cervical area (that part of the chorion adjacent to the opening of the cervix into the uterus). A few foals may reach term and be delivered normally (or be somewhat weaker than normal) because the fungus grows slowly, not involving enough placenta to cause abortion.

Bacterial infections of the placenta may not be sufficiently severe during the acute stage of infection to cause abortion. The body defenses may react sufficiently rapidly and efficiently to destroy the invading organisms and stop the progress of the infection. The pregnancy, then, may carry on to term uneventfully. On the other hand, the inflammation may leave scars after the acute infection has been cleared up. Everyone knows about scars resulting from damage to the skin. Some may not, however, have thought of scars in deeper tissues and organs. The liver, kidney, heart, etc. all can be scarred. The placenta, too, can be scarred. If abortion does not occur during the acute infection, healing and scarring can occur. The scarring renders some areas of the placenta less efficient or totally incapable of carrying out the exchange function. An infection occurs, for example, in the sixth month of pregnancy but is successfully fought off. Scarring occurs, reducing the effective placental exchange area. In the ninth or tenth month of pregnancy, the fetus may run into trouble because of this loss of exchange area, be asphyxiated and die. The infection at six months, then, can be the primary cause, as a result of scarring, of the abortion which occurs at nine months.

Often the first concern with either bacterial or fungal infections of the fetus or placenta is the type of organism involved. In fact, it really doesn't make much difference! Virtually any organism normally found in the mare's environment can enter the uterus, set up infection of the placenta and cause abortion. In fact one often finds several bacteria (and maybe an odd fungus or two) growing on the placenta. The important question is not *which* organisms so much as how they gain admission to the uterine incubator. The answer to that simple question, however, is far from clear.

Present evidence indicates that most infections of the fetus and placenta gain entrance to the pregnant uterus through the cervix in the same way that infection enters the nonpregnant uterus. Years ago, it was thought that infection entering at the time of breeding was all-important. It is quite unreasonable, however, that bacteria entering the uterus at the time of breeding would lie in the uterus for a number of months before starting to infect. Positive evidence that the organism enters close to the time of actual abortion has come forth in recent years. Veterinarians have noted that the cervix of a mare may open during pregnancy and then close again. Normally the cervix should be tightly closed throughout pregnancy, forming a tight seal against the entrance of any foreign material into the uterus. When the cervix opens, even for a brief period, bacteria can enter the uterus. The chorial-endometrial interface is an ideal culture medium for bacteria and fungi as well as the fetus.

The obvious question is: why does the cervix open? We do not know. We do not know how often this happens, how many mares do it, or why they do it when they do. It does appear, however, that estrogen loosens the cervix while progesterone tightens it, suggesting that fluctuation in the levels of these hormones may be responsible.

EPIZOOTIC ABORTION

There are three major causes of epizootic abortion in mares. Epizootic means that, if one abortion occurs, one expects more abortions caused by the same agent within a short period of time. The first of these epizootic agents is *Salmonella abortus-equi*. This is a bacteria that entered the uterus and caused severe infection of the fetus and placenta, resulting in abortion. The organism could spread from the aborted tissues to other mares, infecting them and causing abortion.

Apparently, however, *S. abortus-equi* has disappeared, or, at least, no longer is able to infect mares. A vaccine was developed which was quite effective in perventing the disease, but it is no longer used because the disease no longer exists. We don't know why it disappeared but can simply be thankful that it did so!

The second type of epizootic abortion, one still very much with us, is *rhinopneumonitis*, also known as virus abortion. There is a long story to tell about this virus, a story made clear largely through the work of a truly unsung hero of the history of the horse, the late Dr. E. R. Doll. His years of painstaking and exacting work at the University of Kentucky elucidated the story of rhinopneumonitis infection as well as hemolytic icterus, arteritis, and many other afflictions of the horse.

Rhinopneumonitis is a virus of the herpes group (the same family of viruses that causes cold sores in humans and coital exanthema in horses). The virus is primarily responsible for disease of the respiratory system. Generally, in the autumn, groups of foals will go through a period of "colds" (eloquently known among horsemen as the "snots"). The foals run fevers, go off feed for a day or two, and develop a copious, watery nasal discharge. The virus, traveling about in the air, lands on the lining of the nose and throat and begins to invade the cells which comprise that lining. After invasion, the viral particles proliferate (increase in numbers), break out of the originally invaded cells, and move to new cells, spreading the infection. The mucosa (the lining of the nose) reacts to the damage done to the cells by becoming inflamed. Part of the inflammatory reaction is the production of quantities of mucus which coat the lining cells of the mucosa protecting them as well as physically washing virus away. This mucus is the runny nose so obvious to you and the foal.

As a rule, the infection spreads through all the young foals on the farm that have not been exposed to the virus previously. Without complications, the disease quickly runs its course, and the foal returns to normal. Treatment may not be necessary. If the weather is particularly bad, as it tends to be in the autumn, or if the foals are housed under poor, drafty conditions, secondary infection can occur. This will be discussed in detail, in the section on pleuritis but, for now, it can be said that bacteria (particularly streptococci) can enter the nose and set up an infection in areas already damaged by the virus. Bacterial infection induces a purulent inflammatory reaction. Purulent means pus. White blood cells react to the presence of bacteria more strongly than to virus and, entering the nasal cavity, change the watery mucus to a thick, creamy discharge (a purulent discharge). When this occurs the fever persists, the foal becomes sicker and remains sick for a longer time. Antibiotic treatment is now required. Your veterinarian may recommend antibiotics during the first, purely viral, stage of the disease with the objective of heading off or preventing the bacterial, secondary infection. If you practise good management, and the weather is not too abominable, such preventitive antibiotics are not necessary. Here, as elsewhere, the horseman and veterinarian should discuss the situation and decide on the most rational, and least expensive, program for the benefit of the foals.

If a pregnant mare, or any other older horse, is exposed to rhinopenumonitis virus, she will undergo what is known as a subclinical infection. The virus will set up shop in the nose and begin to invade cells, but, since the mare has experienced the virus before, she will have some resistance to the virus. This resistance will be in the form of antibodies which appear in the nose and quickly wipe out the virus and, hence, the infection. Usually the period of infection is very short, and there will be no overt clinical signs that the mare has experienced the disease. She may skip a meal or run a fever for some hours, but this is usually overlooked or ignored.

That seemed nice and easy, didn't it? There is, however, that short period while the virus is invading the cells of the nose, before the antibody arrives. During this brief period, some viral particles may be engulfed by white blood cells. Once engulfed, they will not be harmed by antibody. In some way not understood, these virus-containing white cells circulate through the bloodstream and eventually reach the uterus. Once there, the virus escapes from the white cells, enters the fetus and infects it.

As a rule, the trip from the mare's nose to fetus takes about 30 days. Once in the fetus the virus goes wild, infecting virtually every tissue and soon causing abortion. It is the general rule, then, that the aborting mare was infected with virus about 30 days earlier.

Typically, though not invariably, virus abortion appears in storms, a number of mares aborting within a short period of time. The first mare to abort does not infect the others; rather, all the mares were exposed to virus some time previously. Once the abortion storm begins, then, it is too late to do anything about it.

Why don't all mares abort? The problem is quite complicated and poorly understood. The white cells containing the virus may be trapped in the spleen or elsewhere and never get to the uterus. Some mares will have greater quantities of antibody than others and will kill off the virus before it can hide in the white cells. Some mares may simply not be as good antibody producers as others and, therefore, less able to kill off virus. The more exposures the mare has had to virus in previous years, the less chance, on average, that she will abort when exposed anew. Apparently, repeated exposure to virus tends to keep the antibody system on its toes, ready to respond quickly to virus invasion. It is not uncommon for older mares on a farm not to abort while the young mares, less experienced with the virus, do abort. Complete and permanent immunity seems to be impossible, however, as the degree of resistance varies from one horse to another.

Control of virus abortion must be considered on a farm to farm basis. If a farm is isolated, with little or no traffic of horses, the risk of introducing virus and causing abortion is small. Young horses, in particular, returning from shows and the racetrack can transport the virus and introduce it to the pregnant mares. Like many other respiratory viruses, rhino-pneumonitis has the best chance of causing trouble, starting infection, in animals that are being moved, stressed and crowded together. It is common for abortion storms to be initiated by animals that have been shipped to the farm and/or have been through sales arenas. This point cannot be overemphasized. Respiratory diseases are most common and serious in stressed, crowded animals. Outbreaks of "snots" in foals, for example, are less common and severe if the foals are not overcrowded in poorly ventilated barns (and many barns are poorly ventilated). In the wild, mares and foals have large areas over which to move and crowd together only for defense. If man insists on crowding a number of animals into a small area, outbreaks of respiratory infection are inevitable.

Sales barns are a singular source of virus infections of all types. Horses from different areas are brought together and pass their viruses around. An animal resistant to a strain of virus indigenous to his or her home area

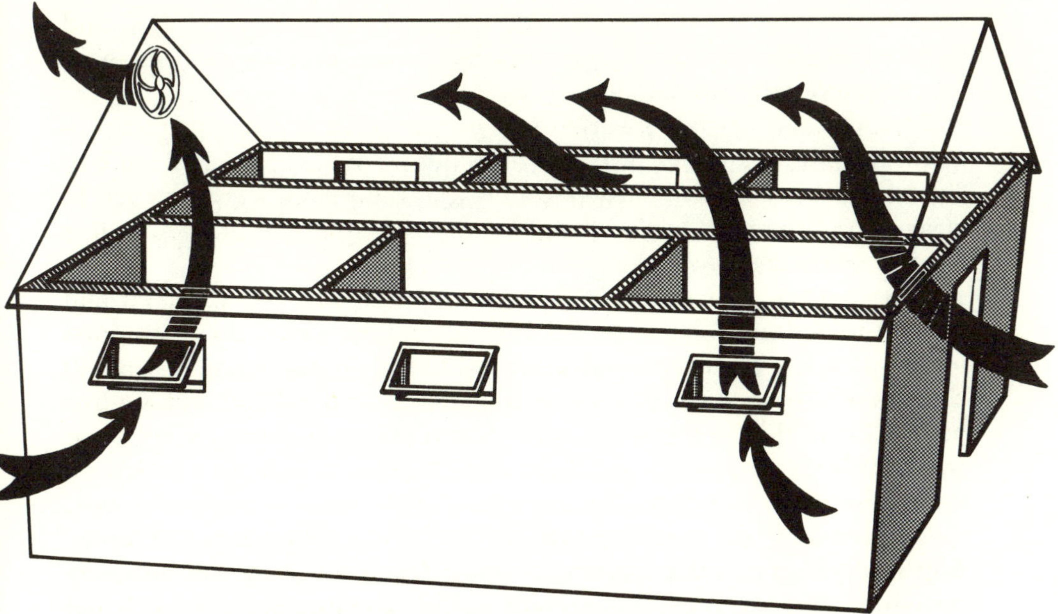

Fig. 7 Some suggestions for proper barn ventilation. Air entering doors and windows is drawn from each individual stall and exhausted above. The air does not travel from stall to stall, possibly spreading airborne infection from one horse to another.

may well become infected with another strain of the same virus brought to the sale barn by an animal from another area.

Proper ventilation of sales and other barns is of great importance because, obviously, we are going to crowd horses together for economic reasons. Figure 7 indicates at least some of the essentials. The flow of air should be uniform and even and not go from horse to horse. In the wide open spaces there is less problem, since most viruses (specifically rhinopneumonitis) cannot travel more than a hundred yards before being killed by the drying effects of air movement and sunlight. In a barn, however, the virus can move considerable distances and stay alive because the air is humid, and there is little or no direct sunlight. Barns are a necessary evil, and the less evil we make them the better.

It must surely be a fool's game to buy mares in foal and sheer idiocy to buy them at an auction barn! If one must buy a mare in foal, he should leave her at the farm where she has been living and ship her after foaling. Pregnant mares should probably not be shipped after the 4th to 5th month. The reason is that rhinopneumonitis virus does not seem to reach or infect the fetus before about the 6th month. This is not invariable, but it is true that most virus abortions occur after the 6th month. After 5 months, then, leave the mare where she is and don't bring in any strange horses to visit her!

We have left to consider the use of vaccines in preventing storms of virus abortion. The oldest vaccine, still in use, was developed for a planned infection program by Dr. Doll. The virus was modified by passing it serially through young hamsters so that the virulence of the virus increased for the hamster but decreased (but did not disappear entirely) for the horse. (Virulence is the ability of the virus to establish an infection.) This modified virus was sprayed into the pregnant mares' noses in midsummer and early fall, setting up a limited infection before the 6th month of pregnancy. This exposure boosted the antibody levels, so that there would be enough antibody on the scene and ready to go to work if wild virus should come along.

The spraying has to be repeated every year because antibody activity decreases very rapidly after exposure to either modified or wild virus. This plan, while not 100% effective against abortion in a given mare, is most effective in preventing storms of abortion and consequent large economic losses.

Another vaccine is now available which, not being live, can be administered at any time. The Doll virus was very risky to use after the 6th month of gestation because it could cause abortion in some mares. At present, the value of this new vaccine is not completely clear. It apparently does no harm, but there is insufficient information to say that it is as good as or better than the live virus vaccine. Time must tell.

The third cause of epizootic abortion in mares is *viral arteritis*. This unusual disease appears to cause abortion accidentally during its infrequent appearances in the United States. To date, outbreaks of the disease have occurred primarily on Standardbred farms, and antibodies detectable by laboratory methods are widespread in the Standardbred horse population. This is evidence of widespread and continuous exposure of these horses to virus. Such evidence of exposure in other horse breeds has so far not been forthcoming. The ecology of the disease is not clear at present, but, thankfully, it is not very common.

Animals of all ages are susceptible. The clinical signs are high fever, loss of appetite, stocking up of all four legs and the under surface of the belly. Close examination will usually show an intense, brick-red discoloration of the conjunctivae of the eyes and other mucous membranes. There will be an effusion (pouring out) of fluid into the chest cavity. In the naturally occurring disease, these clinical signs gradually abate, and the animal returns slowly to normal. If sufficient amounts of virus are given experimentally, however, the horse will die. If there are pregnant mares on the farm, and they become infected, there will be abortions. It is not completely clear whether the abortions are the direct result of viral invasion of the fetus (as with rhinopneumonitis) or simply the result of the severe, life-endangering illness of the mare. Certainly the virus can be isolated from the fetus, but this is not proof that it directly killed the fetus.

The outbreak is usually confined to one farm and runs its course within a few weeks. Almost all, if not all, pregnant mares will abort. There is some evidence that the administration of large quantities of steroids will shorten the course of the natural disease and prevent death in experimental cases. There is no evidence the steroids will prevent the abortions, but they could be worth trying.

There is a vaccine for this disease, but it is not being used because outbreaks have been so infrequent. Experimental studies indicate it is effective and will be available for use if large-scale outbreaks of the disease should ever occur.

OTHER CAUSES OF ABORTION

As mentioned earlier, the mare sick with arteritis infection might abort with or without the virus being directly responsible for fetal death, and that idea needs to be pursued a bit farther. A mare may abort a decomposed fetus several days after an attack of colic or other "illness" no matter what its cause. It is certainly true that impending abortion with uterine contractions and the pains originating therefrom can be the cause of colicky signs. It is also true, at least theoretically, that a severe case of true colic associated with upset of the vascular system (shock in other words) can result in decreased blood flow to the uterus and result in asphyxiation of the fetus. Some abortions, then, which cannot be defined, may be the result of illness of the mare. While unproven, the concept needs to be kept in mind.

Trauma and shipping are often cited as causes of abortion in mares. This is largely wishful thinking. A kick seems less frightening than a virus! One would have to traumatize a mare almost unto to death before abortion would occur. The great danger of shipping mares in foal is not shipping *per se* but the exposure, as already discussed, to rhinopneumonitis virus. Obviously, long, exhausting trips without rest, food and water can be detrimental to a pregnant mare, as to any other animal, but there is no direct relationship to abortion.

Abortion can be the result of congenital malformations of the fetus which are so extensive that intra-uterine life is impossible. Such malformations are not that common in horses, however, and represent a small percentage of abortions.

A twisted umbilical cord is often cited as a cause of abortion. This is a myth. The umbilical cord is normally twisted and, after death of the fetus, blood may pool in the cord and look quite nasty although it had nothing whatsoever to do with abortion. Rarely, the umbilical cord may wrap around a leg or the neck shutting off blood flow to that part, killing the part. With the death of a part, the whole fetus dies and is aborted.

Having considered these known or suspected causes of abortion still leaves thirty to forty per cent of all abortions to be explained. Pathological examination reveals only that the fetus and placenta are decomposed, and no significant lesions or infectious agents can be found. All we can do is say: "Cause of abortion undetermined." Sorry, but a fact is a fact.

One nice feature of such unknowns is that they are all single mare problems. So far, there have been no epizootic forms of abortion for which the cause is not known. One can worry about the one mare that has aborted, but need not worry about the rest of the mares! Small compensation perhaps but compensation in any case.

3
FOALING

We move on now to the culmination of pregnancy, foaling time. When is that? The average of 333 days (range 315 to 350) is usually given. Each mare, however, is her own boss and will do things in her own way and at her own time. Foaling time for the maiden mare can usually only be approximated. Older mares are more reliable, tending to foal at the same time, year after year. There is a strong genetic component since daughters will tend to do the same as their mothers, though not always!

Most mares foal at night. The reason for this is unknown, although it probably goes back to the wild state. The mare is virtually defenseless while foaling and could best hide her vulnerability in darkness.

How does one know that a mare is preparing to foal? Once again, knowing that particular mare's habits is the best guide. Generally, however, the mare will begin to bag up, the udder enlarging rapidly with a waxy secretion appearing at the end of the teats. There will be a perceptible loosening of the tissues in the perineal area (beneath the tail, around the vulva). There may be some periods of discomfort, groaning and even colicky pains which appear for short periods and then go away. Keep cool! When the mare is ready, she will lie down, roll, get up, and lie down again, repeating this process a number of times. Often she will look around at her sides because of mild pain and the sensation of the uterine contractions (what's going on back there!). Finally, she will lie down and begin to strain heavily with heaving contractions of the belly muscles. Shortly, a red sack may appear at the vulva. It quickly ruptures, and a flood of fluid (the allantoic fluid) runs out. The red sack (the chorion) often ruptures inside the vagina and will not be seen. A few more powerful heaves, and a white sack may appear. This is the amnion and, again, it may rupture inside, pouring out the amniotic fluid. Quickly, since the foal is now in the birth canal (the mare's pelvis), the two forefeet and the nose appear and, with a few more big heaves, the foal is out on the ground. That is normal, more or less, though I emphasize again that the mare is an individual and may vary the pattern considerably.

What can go wrong? Many things, and we shall consider first what man does wrong in his efforts to help the mare do something that she knows more about than he does!

While maiden mares may lose their cool (after all it is the first time!), older mares almost invariably know what they're about and get on with it. If one wishes the mare to foal in a box stall which is, in fact, not the best (a nice, clean paddock with room and privacy is best), the stall should be prepared with clean bedding, and the mare moved in some time before the anticipated foaling date. The mare must become acquainted with her surroundings, have no fear of them, and be given privacy. The latter is most important. As foaling time approaches she should be checked regularly and quietly with minimum noise and lights. Preferably the foaling attendant should be someone the mare knows well.

When delivery begins, the attendant may quietly enter the stall and wait a moment for the mare to become aware of his presence. He will have thoroughly cleaned and scrubbed his hands and arms before entering the stall. Approaching the mare carefully and quietly, he should slip one hand into the vagina and feel for the two feet and nose. If they cannot be located with the hand inserted about one foot, the attendant should leave the stall and wait. Try again a short while later. When both feet and the nose can be felt, he should leave the stall. Everything is coming along properly. If only one foot, no nose or something other than two feet and nose are presenting, the veterinarian should be called immediately. Something may be wrong and it is best to have the veterinarian on his way, just in case. From the start of labor to delivery is usually only 30 minutes, more or less, so that there isn't much time to stand around wondering whether to do something.

I am, obviously, not talking here to experienced foaling men and night watchmen. It would be presumptious of me to tell those experts how to go about a job that they have been through many more times than I. Incidentally, if you live near such a person, a large horse farm, a friendly discussion with those men will be more than worth your time.

If no veterinarian is available, here are a few guidelines to follow:

1) If one foot and the nose are presenting, it is safe to reach carefully into the vagina to search for the other foot. Usually, it is flexed or folded back. The foot can be pulled toward the midline, then back and out.
2) If only the head is presenting, both front feet are folded back. They must be found and pulled out, one at a time.

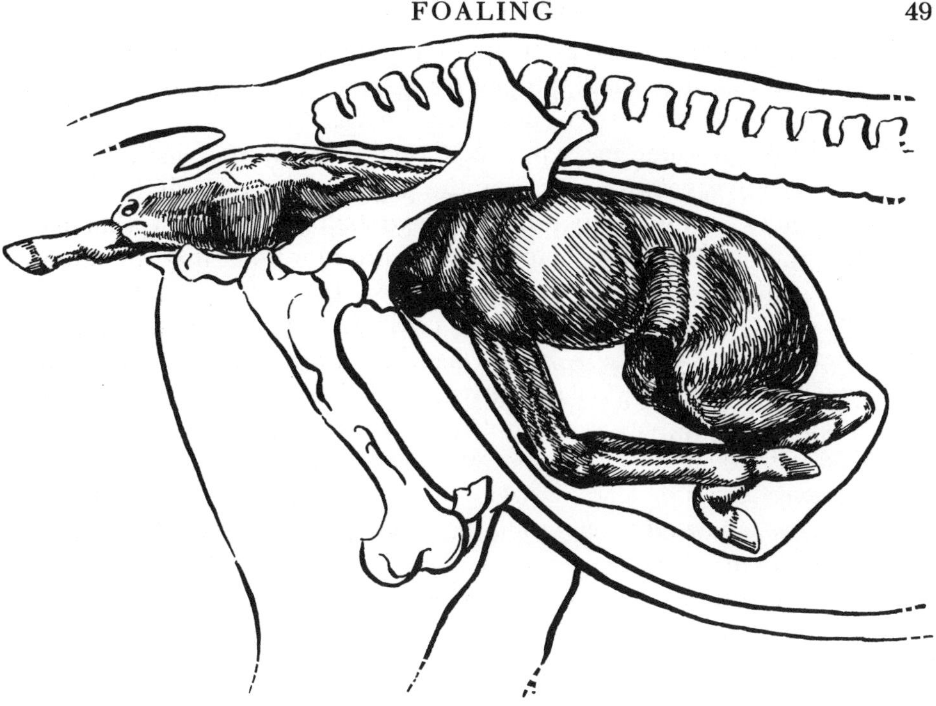

Fig. 8 Abnormal presentation of the foal with one leg retained.

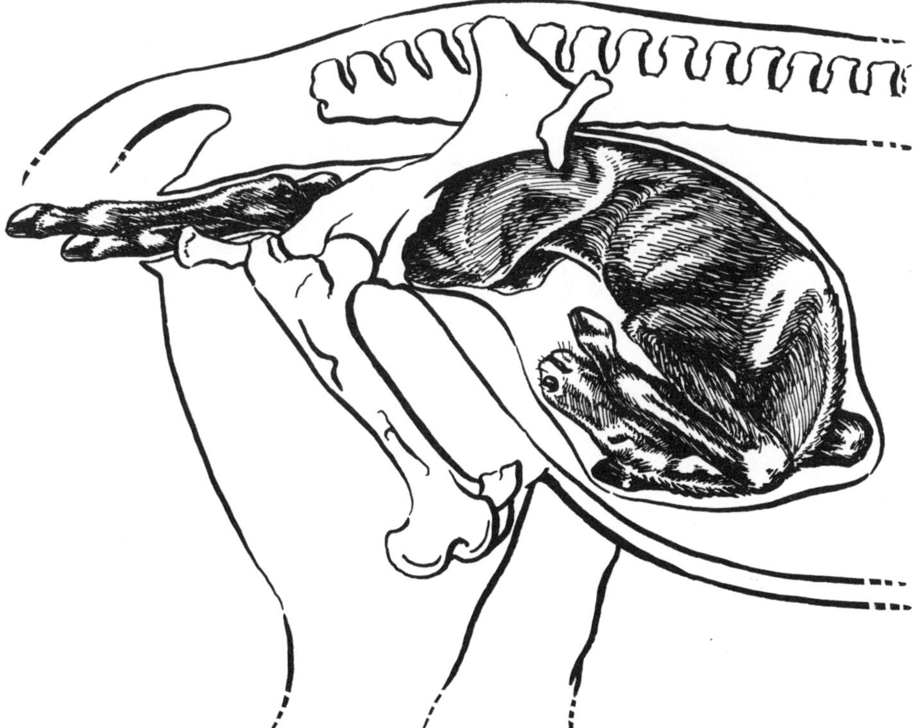

Fig. 9 Abnormal presentation of the foal with both forelegs presenting but the head retained.

3) If both front feet are presenting, but head is not, search for the head, grasp the lower jaw, and gradually work the head back and out.

With any of these maneuvers, the mare will probably strain. The search for parts of the foals body should be done between the heaves of the mare. It will be easier, and the straightening of body parts can be accomplished more readily.

Often, it will be necessary to push the foal back into the mare, between straining periods. This should be done in cases where more room is needed to pull out a leg or a head. The more room one has, the better off he will be. After the foal has been pushed back in, the mare will probably push it right back out again.

4) The rear feet and tail presenting is a dangerous situation. The umbilical cord is compressed in the pelvis of the mare and the oxygen supply is, therefore, cut off. If the feet are out, they should be gotten hold of through steady and continuous pulling straight back. As soon as the foal's rearquarters clear the vulva, the direction of pull should be adjusted from straight back to the direction of the mare's rear feet. This gradual, circular

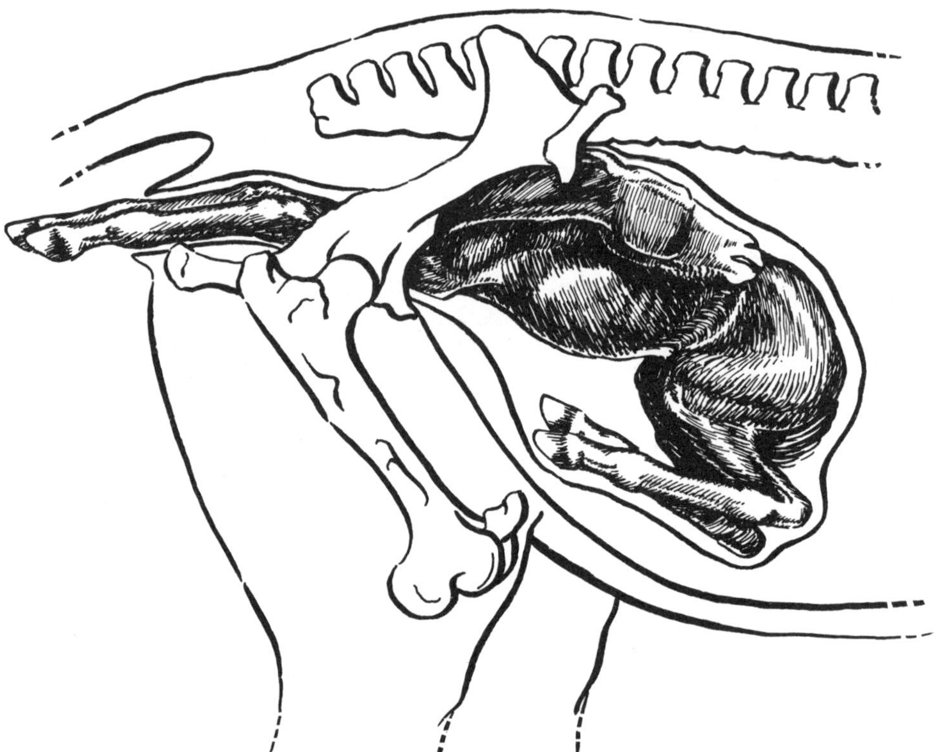

Fig 10   **Abnormal presentation of the foal with the rear feet and tail presenting.**

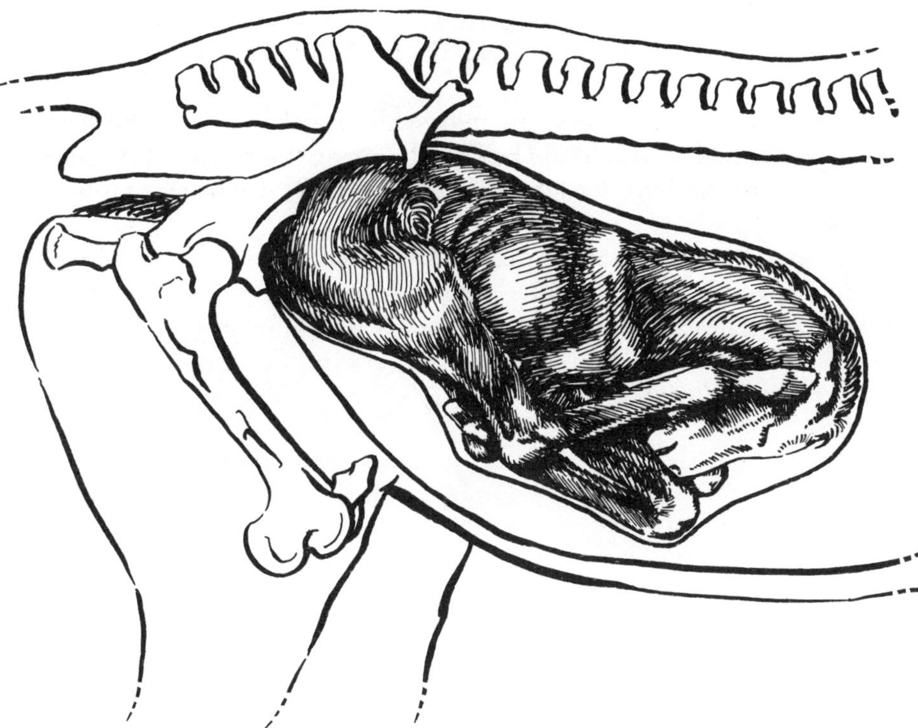

Fig. 11 Breech presentation. The tail only is presenting with the rear feet retained.

change of direction conforms to the matural shape of the mare's pelvis and makes delivery much easier. Unfortunately, even with prompt assistance, such foals are often suffocated in the birth canal and stillborn.

5) If the tail but no feet are presenting, it may be possible to feel only the hocks. The foal, then, *must* be pushed back in as far as possible and an attempt made to locate and pull out one foot and then the other. This presentation is the most difficult to correct, and the foal is almost always dead. The primary concern, in this case, is to save the mare.

6) A large part of the red sack, the allantochorion, breaks off and comes out before the foal's forefeet and head. The foal has lost a large portion of the placenta together with its oxygen supply and will soon be suffocating. The forelegs, in this case, should be grasped firmly and a steady traction exerted. As soon as the foal's chest clears, the pull should be redirected toward the mare's rear feet as described above.

Obviously, there are other things that can go wrong. All four feet may be presenting with no head. This is a disastrous presentation. The foal

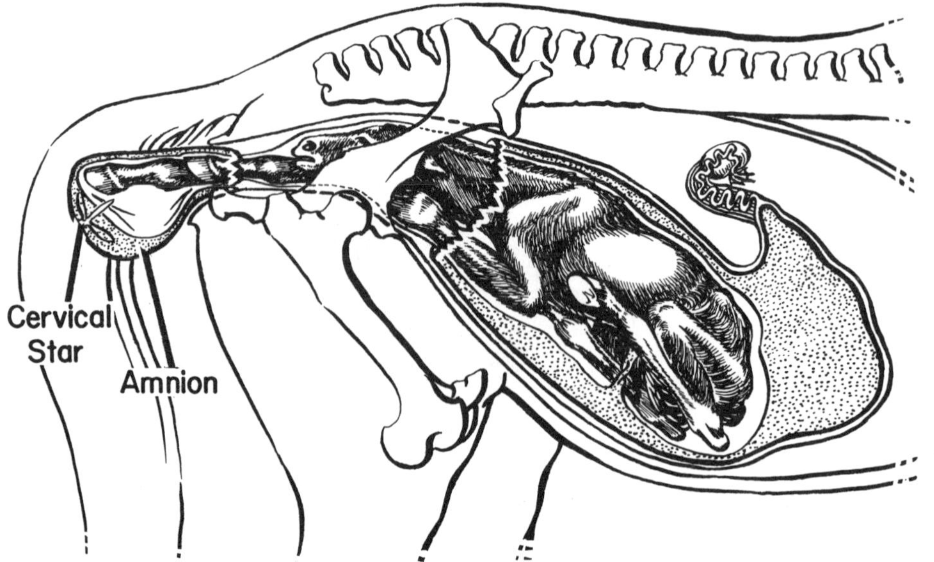

Fig. 12   Number 6 in the text. The allantochorion has broken off abnormally instead of through the cervical star as it should.

may be upside down. If these or other malpositions cannot be corrected, the mare should be disturbed. She should be walked in order to interrupt the delivery process until professional help can arrive. Walking, also, may allow the foal to straighten itself out, so that the delivery can proceed.

Maiden mares may panic and race about the stall. The attendant may be able to quiet the mare. If this does not work, it may be best to let the maiden into a small paddock with older mares in adjacent paddocks (this should be arranged for before hand, just in case). The nickering horse talk of the old "pros" may be all the frightened mare needs to calm her. In any case, there will be more room and less chance of the half-delivered foal being slammed against the walls of the stall.

This is not meant to create a panicky situation. Most mares will do the job on their own in fine style if there is not too much human help. The nearest veterinarian should be notified when foaling is anticipated, however. If the mare is sutured, he will come along a few days before and open the vulva to avoid tearing when the foal is delivered. He is also alerted to the possibility of a late night foaling call.

When the foal has been born, there may be membranes draped over its head. They should be pulled off and then the mare and foal should be left alone. If the mare is lying down, the umbilical cord will usually remain

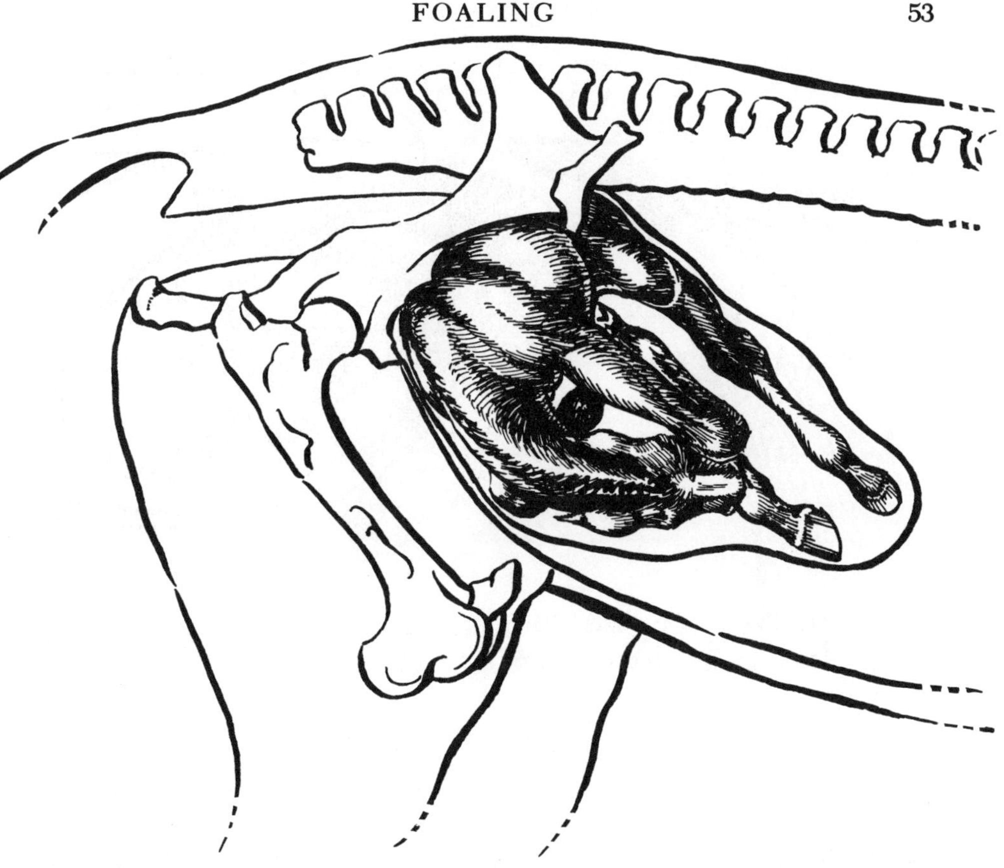

Fig. 13   Transverse presentation. The foal cannot be delivered this way and must be repositioned to a head or tail first presentation.

attached to the foal. The placenta is still in the uterus and will be delivered in due course. The placenta will contract after birth and squeeze several pints of blood into the foal. The cord should not be broken before the foal has received this blood. Usually, the foal will break the cord in its struggles to stand, within 15 minutes after birth. If, as rarely happens, the cord does not break, the veterinarian should be allowed to do it. He can detect the natural stricture in the cord an inch or so from the foal's belly and pull on the cord until it breaks just at the proper place. The cord should not be tied off. Only fantastic bleeding can justify tying.

THE POSTPARTURIENT MARE

We now consider what can go wrong with the mare during and

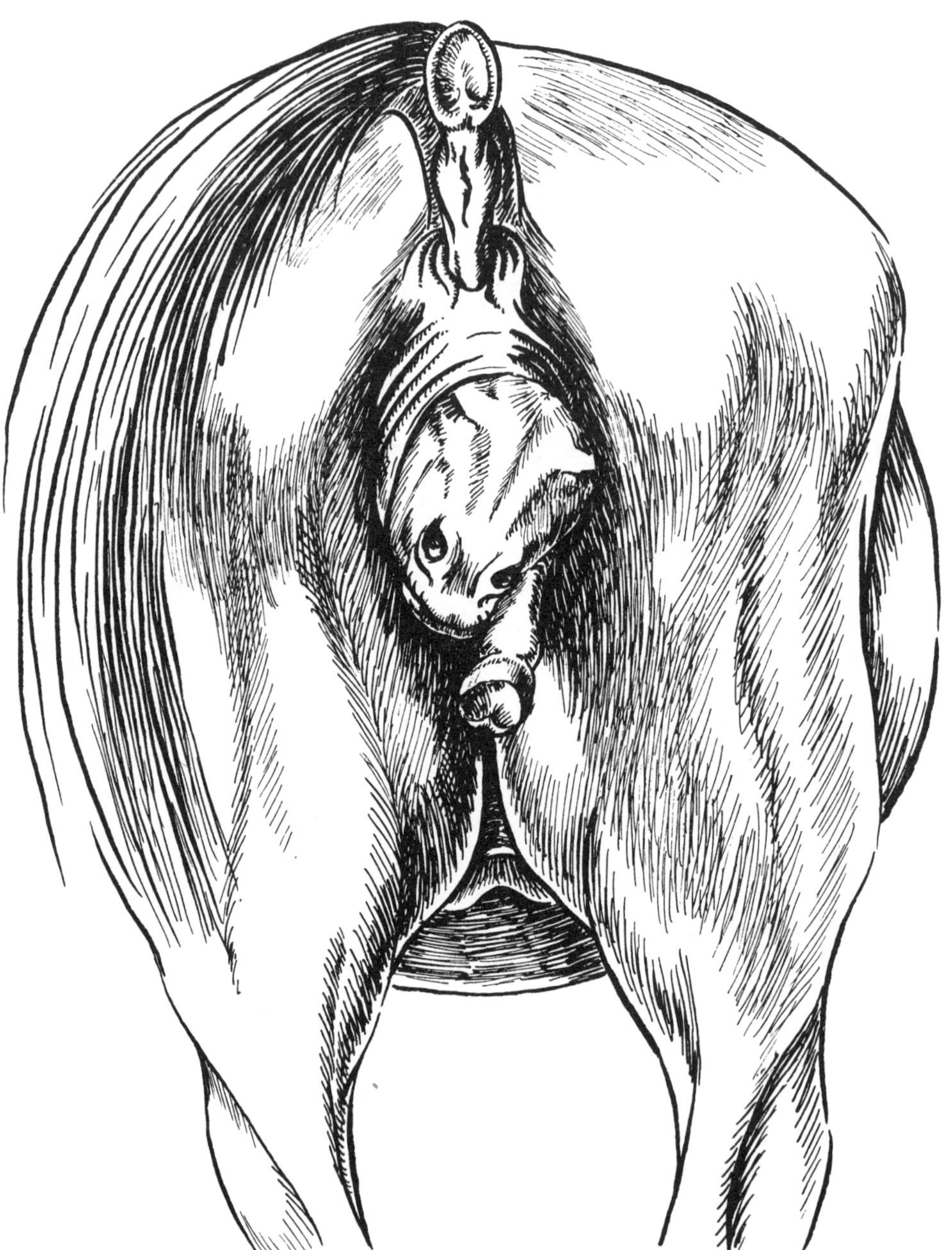

Fig. 14 Rearview of mare delivering foal with one of the foal's feet tearing through the wall of the vagina and the rectum.

immediately after foaling. The force and speed of the foaling process predisposes the mare to a variety of traumatic injuries. Among the more obvious are tearing of the cervix, vaginal wall and vulva. As a rule such tears heal without untoward aftereffects. Occasionally, however, rather severe damage is done, and considerable scarring and distortion may occur during the healing process. While the scarring may not interfere with subsequent conception, it can be real factor in future foalings. Trauma to the vulva and vagina can often be surgically corrected with reasonable expectation of good functional results. Unfortunately, severe lacerations usually involve the cervix, and surgical reconstruction of this area is difficult and often without good functional results.

More devastating injuries, almost peculiar to the mare, are, once again, the result of the rapid and powerful nature of the foaling process. One foot of the foal may break through the upper wall of the vagina and tear into the rectum which lies just above it. As the foal is driven out the foot comes along, tearing out the roof of the vagina and the floor of the rectum, the end result being a common opening between the two. This condition is, for some reason, known as "gill-flirted". While a horrid looking mess, these tears can be nicely repaired once the initial swelling and inflammation have subsided. These *recto-vaginal fistulas* can be variable in size. Not all are caused by the mechanism described. Delayed delivery with continuous pressure being exerted by the foal on the rectal and vaginal tissues may cause ischemic necrosis. Ischemia is the loss of blood supply to the area as result of pressure squeezing the blood vessels shut. Necrosis, death of the tissues, is the result of the closing down of the blood supply. Often, the fistula resulting from such pressure necrosis is quite small and only detected by careful vaginal examination. A fistula may be suspected if there is persistent vaginal inflammation (bacteria from the rectum dripping into and infecting the vagina) and/or fecal material in the vagina and running from the vulva. Such fistulas must be repaired, no matter how small, or the mare's reproductive tract will be continually reinfected by fecal bacteria.

A more devastating accident is a tremendous build-up of pressure in the rectum as the foal is passing through the pelvis. Such pressures can, though fortunately rarely do, burst the mare's rectum like a balloon. When that happens, fecal material is spread throughout the tissues of the pelvis, and severe infection develops. Heroic treatment is necessary and may be frustrated because of abscess formation. If the rectum ruptures within the abdominal cavity, fatal, usually untreatable, peritonitis quickly follows. Surgical repair can be attempted, but the infection moves rapidly and can rarely be contained.

Also rare, happily, is the turning of the mare's cecum (part of the large intestine) into the pelvis as the foal is trying to pass through the pelvic canal. Again, a balloon effect occurs, and the cecum ruptures within the abdominal cavity with peritonitis the quick and fatal result.

Older mares (10 years or more) may bleed severely and fatally after an apparently normal foaling. This problem is peculiar to the mare, probably because we breed mares to much more advanced ages than other species. Within an hour or two after an uneventful foaling the mare begins to tremble and sweat profusely. The mucous membranes are very pale, and the pulse is fast, thin and weak. The rectal temperature may be lower than normal. After a few hours these signs may abate, and the mare may seem to be recovering. Suddenly all the previous signs reappear in more severe form, and the mare quickly dies. What has happened is that a major artery supplying the uterus has been torn during foaling. The

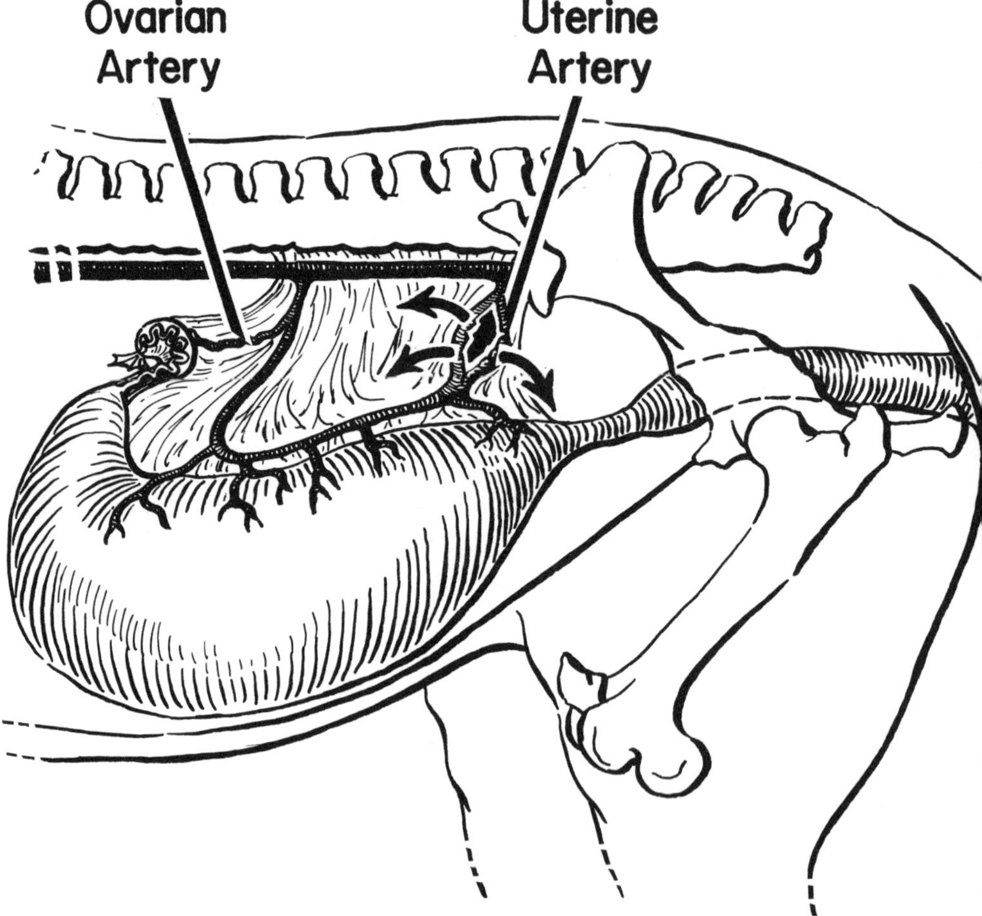

Fig. 15   Rupture and bleeding from the uterine artery in the postparturient older mare. The ovarian artery may also tear.

uterine artery is most commonly affected. Blood pours out of the artery between the two sheets of tissue which make up the broad ligament, an outfolding of the peritoneum which holds the uterus in place. When the bleeding into the space formed by the two sheets of the broad ligament occurs, the first set of clinical signs appears. These signs are those of hemorrhagic shock, a drop in blood pressure throughout the body as a result of extensive loss of blood. If the tear in the artery is not too large, the blood may clot and the bleeding stops. If the tear is sufficiently large (and it usually is) the large mass of blood (hematoma) will split open one of the sheets of the broad ligament, and blood will pour unhindered into the abdominal cavity. This sudden spilling of blood precipitates the second set of signs of profound hemorrhagic shock, and the mare is soon dead.

There is no treatment. The animal should be put in or kept in her stall, darkened and quiet, and left strictly alone, hoping that her blood pressure will stay low and clotting will occur. While surgical repair has been considered, it is not feasible. Bleeding is massive from the beginning, and it is difficult to identify, even at postmortem examination, the vessel which is involved. Blood transfusions and coagulant drugs simply do not work. Even if clotting occurs and the mare survives, it is likely that she will bleed again at a subsequent foaling. The system is wearing out, and the bleeding is the sign that the reproductive life of the mare is nearly at an end.

A few mares may bleed to death during the seventh month of pregnancy because of rupture of the ovarian artery, in the absence of any sign of foaling. Such mares are always very old, and the weight and movement of the fetus within the uterus are sufficient to tear the aging ovarian artery.

From the pathological evidence it seems clear that there is a gradual accumulation of wear and tear damage to the arteries of the uterus with each succeeding pregnancy. Eventually, a sufficient amount of scarring and weakening of the arterial wall occurs, so that the normal activity of foaling can tear the vessel. The uterine arteries change size remarkably during pregnancy and carry a large volume of blood under high pressure, predisposing them to wear and tear changes earlier than other vessels in the body.

The mare usually delivers the placenta within a half hour of foaling. Leaving the umbilical cord attached to the foal will help delivery of the contracting placenta by simply physical pulling. The uterus also contracts (called "involution" of the uterus) helping to expel the placenta. These uterine involuting contractions can be quite strong and may cause the mare to show signs similar to colic (discomfort, looking around at the side).

Once the placenta has been delivered it should be carefully laid out on a smooth surface and examined to be sure that it is all present. It is worthwhile to have the veterinarian conduct this examination. If even a small piece is left in the uterus, it will undergo decomposition and may precipitate an attack of postparturient founder (laminitis). While laminitis is always bad, the postparturient form is absolutely the worst. It should be avoided if possible because it is so very difficult to treat satisfactorily. Apropos of this, the placenta should *not* be pulled out as soon as it appears or cut off because it is unsightly, but should be allowed to hang. Its own weight will help to assure a smooth, steady separation from the uterus and minimize the chances for a small piece to be torn loose and left in the uterus.

It is inevitable that bacteria will enter the uterus during and immediately after foaling. The healthy mare will clear them within 48 hours of foaling, on average. There may be a reddish, thick, fluid discharge from the vulva for a few days. This is blood, mucus, and damaged endometrial lining which is being sloughed out and is quite normal.

The question of breeding back on the foal heat, that estrus which occurs 9-10 days after foaling, has been long and arduously debated. If the mare has foaled and cleaned (delivered the placenta) normally, the discharges clear up quickly, and the veterinarian's examination indicates that she is not infected and not bruised or torn badly, then it is perfectly reasonable to breed her. If any of these conditions are not met, however, then it is best for the mare's sake, to wait until the next heat period.

4

THE NEWBORN FOAL

The foal may be born dead or alive. Often, however, it is not clear why the foal has failed to make the transition from intrauterine to extrauterine life. What is truly amazing, considering the complexity of the process, is that so many do make the transition, not that a few don't.

Most stillborns submitted for pathological examination show clear signs of asphyxiation (suffocation). They died of lack of oxygen at some point during the changeover from the placental oxygen supply to obtaining their own oxygen from the air through their lungs. This is called *neonatal asphyxia* (suffocation of the newborn).

1) Asphyxiation may occur because, for some unknown reason, the placenta separated from the endometrium too long before delivery was completed. This can be determined with some degree of certainty by examination of the placenta but is a task for the expert.
2) Part of the body of the placenta may break off and be delivered before the foal, as described earlier.
3) A fungus or, less commonly, a bacteria may have infected the placenta (usually the body of the placenta). While the damage (loss of exchange surface) was not sufficient to kill the foal and cause abortion, it has so reduced the oxygen exchange that the foal simply did not have enough reserves, enough strength, to undergo the normal rigors of the foaling process.
4) Delayed delivery is probably the commonest cause of neonatal asphyxia and is, perhaps, the most difficult to understand or clearly define at post-mortem examination. The foal may show only nonspecific signs of asphyxia-tion. When the attendants have observed the foaling and know (and admit) that there was a delay while a leg was straightened or a breech delivery

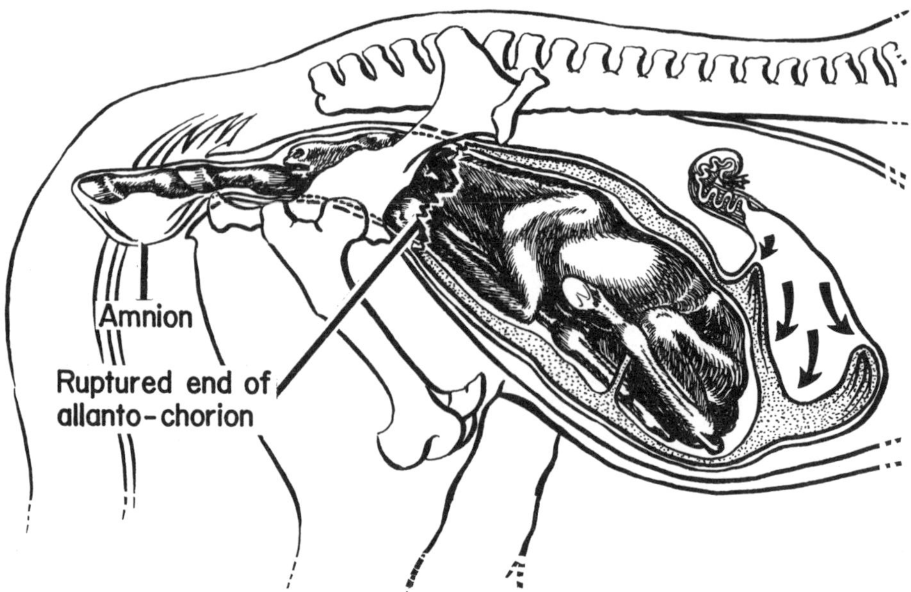

Fig. 16　In this schematic illustration premature separation of a part of the allantochorion is shown, indicated by the arrows.

affected, there is no difficulty in understanding what went wrong. Without such a history, the determination of the cause of asphyxiation can be difficult. In the simplest case, there may be several broken ribs which have stuck into or torn the heart and/or lungs. From the location of these fractures it seems that the elbow of the foal was pressed or jammed against the ribs, breaking the ribs while the foal was within the mare's pelvis. This could occur because the forelegs were not fully extended as the foal passed through the nonyielding pelvis of the mare. Also, if the forelegs are not fully extended, there may be a delay in delivery, and the foal suffocates during this delay, with or without broken ribs.

If such an obvious cause is not apparent, examination of the shoulder joints may provide an answer. With delay and jamming in the birth canal there will be pressure on and frank bleeding into the shoulder joints. I have seen a sufficient number of foals, dead on arrival, with a definite history of delayed delivery to be quite sure that such bleeding into the joints is virtually *prima facie* evidence of delay. Establishing this diagnosis does not help the dead foal, obviously, but having an answer is at least some compensation.

Broken ribs are not always fatal. The foal may appear quite normal and the breaks detectable only by careful palpation of the chest wall in the region of the elbow. If such fractures are detected, it is the usual practise to limit the foal's exercise for some days to a week or more while healing occurs. It is quite common to find a number of fractures at the junctions of the ribs and sternum (costochondral fractures). They are of little or no significance and heal rapidly and uneventfully.

Foals born dead should always be examined promptly by the veterinarian or the laboratory. There is at least one condition, fortunately quite rare, which justifies such examination. The mare's cervix opens some hours, at least, prior to delivery and a bacteria, *Escherichia coli*, may enter and infect the foal. The foal will be born dead or die within a few hours. The postmortem will show severe hemorrhagic inflammation of the intestinal tract. Usually the endometrium of the uterus is infected as well, and this may lead to an extensive and life-endangering infection of the whole uterus (metritis). The dead foal's intestine provides the clue that the mare may have such a severe and potentially fatal infection of the uterus which should be promptly and thoroughly treated. There are a few other bacteria which can do this as well, but *E. coli* is the most important.

Occasionally, for reasons unknown in most cases, a mare will foal earlier than normal. Such a *premature foal* may be the result of a placental disease and the premature foaling, then, is actually a late abortion. The premature foal, explained or unexplained, usually dies sooner or later. From the evidence available such foals do not have the lung disease which so frequently afflicts the premature human infant (so-called hyaline membrane disease). Rather, the premature foal's primary problem appears to be that the intestinal tract does not work properly. While the intestine may be able to move, contracting and relaxing, it seems unable to do so in a coordinated manner which permits the expelling of gas and meconium and the normal movement of ingesta along the tract. Gas can accumulate and precipitate rather marked colicky pain. If the foal nurses, colic usually follows immediately afterward because of an overfilling of a gut not moving in a coordinated fashion. Drugs do not seem to help this problem. Frequent enemas, mechanically stimulating the large intestine to expell gas, and mild sedation to alleviate the colicky pain seem to be the only treatments available.

While uncommon it is occasionally necessary to perform a caesarian section in order to deliver the foal. Although frequently successful with other species, it is not often so with the mare. The foal may be removed neatly and cleanly, and the mare may recover from the surgery without incident. The foal, however, will not usually survive. If not born dead (asphyxia as result of delayed delivery), it will usually be weak and barely breathing. The foal will probably neither stand nor nurse and can be kept alive only by heroic nursing measures. As with the premature foal the intestinal tract does not function normally. Perhaps the foal needs the stimulation of passing through the mare's pelvis in order to stimulate proper breathing (portions of the lungs usually fail to expand properly in the caesarian foal). What has been said pertains primarily to the light horse breeds. Mixed breds and ponies may be delivered by caesarian with survival of both mare and foal. Whatever the chances for the foal, the caesarian is usually done in order to save the mare when normal delivery is impossible.

The next problem is the vexing one of so-called "dummy" or "sleeper" foals. We have some of the answers but hardly all. Certain foals are born normally and seem to have every right to go on without difficulty. Within a few hours, however, it is apparent that the foal is, like the caesarian foal, floppy, barely alive and unwilling to make any attempt to get up and nurse. Careful examination may reveal evidence of a bacterial infection, but, quite honestly, many of these foals coming to postmortem have no lesions to explain why they died. There has to be a reason; we simply haven't been smart enough to find it. Some do, however, tell their story.

As mentioned previously the mare's cervix opens some time before actual delivery, and bacteria can enter and infect the foal in those last few hours before birth. *E. coli* has been discussed. Two other bacteria, *Shigella* and *Streptococcus*, may be the ones to enter. They may infect and kill the foal before birth, so that it is born dead, or they may infect and still be working on the foal as it is born. The foal may appear normal for some hours, standing and nursing, while the disease is incubating. When the infection is fully developed, the foal collapses, becomes very ill and dies within a matter of hours.

The shigella bacteria is one of the major causes of illness and death of the foal during the first two to three weeks of life. This bacteria is ubiquitous in the horse environment and may infect the foal before birth, as noted, or anytime during the first few weeks of life. After roughly one month, the animal becomes resistant to the disease, why this is so we do not know. Perhaps someone will try to find out. It is known that the foal which receives colostrum (the first, antibody-rich fluid from the mare's udder) is more resistant to shigella infection.

The first signs to alert the horseman to the presence of this infection are: 1) the foal stops nursing (the mare's udder is distended), 2) appears listless or sleepy, and 3) the mucous membranes are redder than normal. There may be diarrhea. The rectal temperature will be higher than normal, and there may be lameness with one or more hot, swollen joints. Note well! The first sign of this infection may be lameness with or without an obviously swollen joint. Horsemen are great believers in trauma, the "kick by the mare," and, unless experienced, think that the foal has been injured. The foal's temperature should be taken and a veterinarian summoned. If it really was a kick (uncommon), the treatment does no

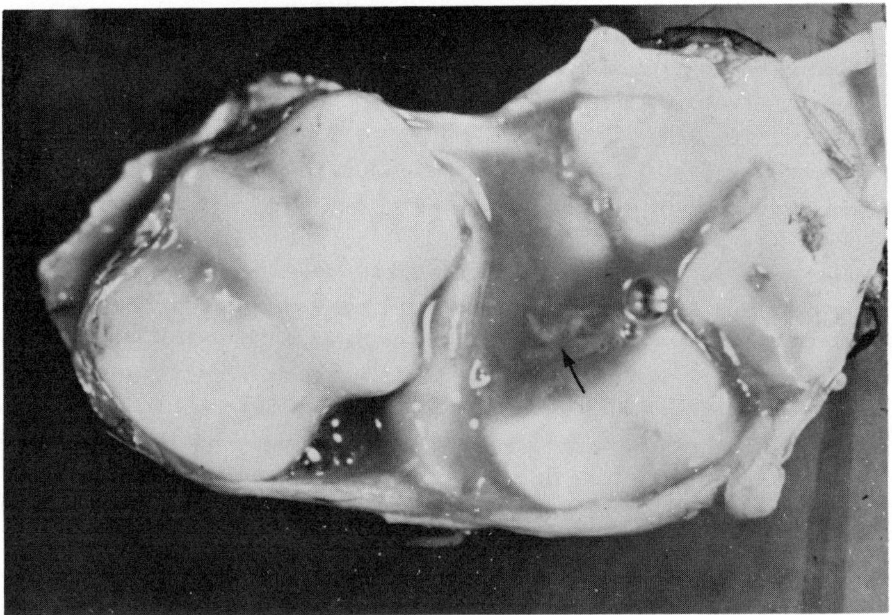

Fig. 17 Photograph of an infected fetlock joint in a young foal. The arrow indicates pus in the joint fluid.

harm, and if it wasn't a kick, the foal's life will be saved. I emphasize this because you do not have much time. Shigella produce an endotoxin, and treatment must be initiated quickly before sufficient toxin has been produced to kill the foal. Full levels of antibiotics are essential and they must be the right kind. A veterinarian will know which antibiotics and combinations should be used in certain areas. Not all antibiotics work equally well in all geographical areas.

Once a great killer, shigella is no longer because of antibiotics. The disease apparently occurs as frequently as it always has, but the foals survive with the help of antibiotics and do not appear as statistics in postmortem surveys and reports.

It has long been axiomatic that the *navel* of the newborn foal must be painted with a disinfectant solution, usually iodine or a similar drug. In fact, one application of such an antiseptic will do little good. It will kill the bacteria present at the time of application but will not kill the bacteria that arrive later. The best navel treatment is a scrupulously clean foaling stall and abundant, uncrowded pasture. Since both of these are rare, one may sluice the navel daily until it begins to dry up and seal off, using a mild, organic iodine solution. Never use strong, alcoholic solutions with the idea of sealing up the navel. Nature designed the navel to weep fluids

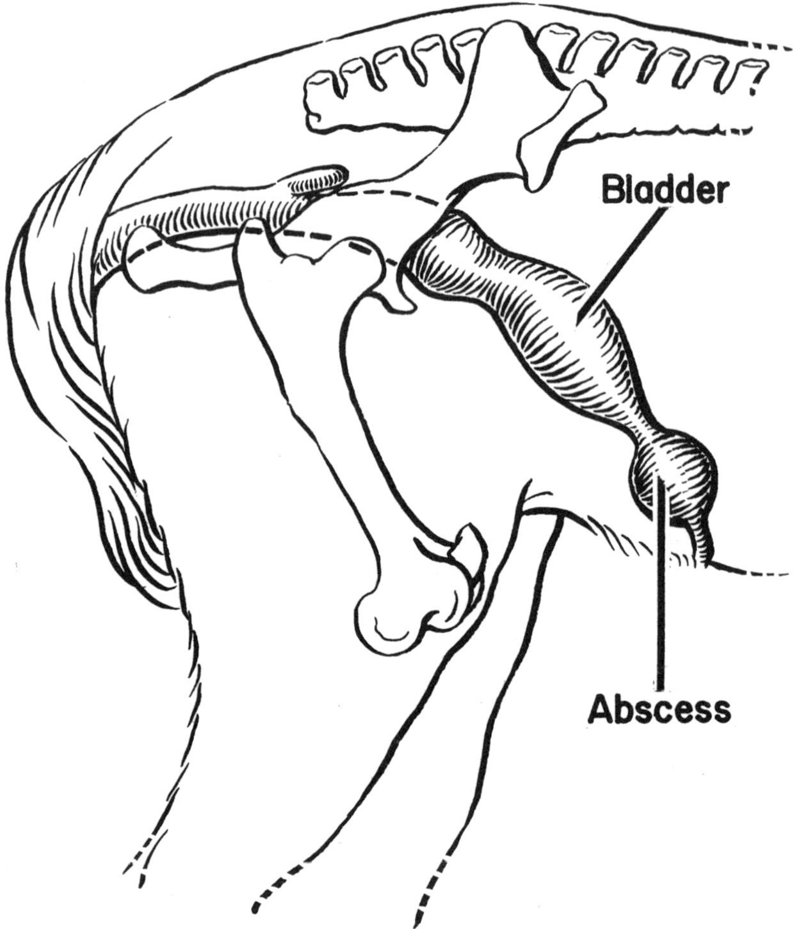

Fig. 18   Schematic side view showing the site of a urachus abscess just above the umbilicus, inside the abdomen.

almost continuously for several days after birth. The weeping washes away bacteria and other foreign matter, helping to keep the navel clean. This is a natural, effective protective mechanism and should not be interfered with. If you do seal the navel too quickly (before it does so spontaneously) bacteria may be sealed in, grow, and cause formation of a so-called urachus abscess inside the foal's belly. That abscess can cause trouble later.

During this same period and continuing until, roughly, two to three months of age, the other major pathogen of the foal (a pathogen is an agent which causes disease), *Streptococcus*, may begin its dirty work. Streptococci, like shigella, are ubiquitous wherever there are horses. They may infect the foal before, during or after birth. The clinical signs may be identical to those of shigella infection. As a rule of thumb, and only that, streptococcal infections do not progress quite as rapidly. Despite that fact, adequate and thorough treatment must be quickly set in motion. Streptococci, again, like shigella, like to infect joints. Unlike shigella, however, streptococci destroy the joint cartilages and may render the foal a permanent cripple. It is important, then, to continue antibiotic treatment for a minimum of one week, or five to six days after all clinical signs have abated, in order to clear all the bacteria from the body. Unless all the bacteria are cleared by adequate treatment recurrence of infection, one joint after another, is to be expected and the foal eventually will be lost.

If adequate treatment has not been carried out, and a joint does flare up, then there is real trouble. The foal must now be treated vigorously and expensively, often for several weeks, in order to eliminate the bacteria in the joints. Even this may not work and heroic and dangerous intravenous injections of large doses of penicillin may become necessary. Each such intravenous injection increases the risk of sudden anaphylactic shock and death. It is better to treat the disease properly the first time.

Certain foals infected with either of these organisms and, indeed, almost any other, may die despite the best efforts and the finest of antibiotics. Why? There are no clear answers in all cases. This may result from the foal simply being weak and improperly equipped to deal with the exigencies of life outside the uterus. The foal was not meant to live. That seems a most unsatisfactory and unscientific thing to say, but it is true.

From other species we know that some individuals are born without the ability to form antibodies. This has been called agammaglobulinemia or hypogammaglobulinemia (these terms mean total or partial lack of gamma globulin, the blood protein of which antibodies are made). The condition is well-known in the human. There is little direct evidence that such inherited defects in the immune mechanism occur in foals with the exception of certain lines of Arabians as will be discussed later. Other components of the defense mechanism may be missing as well as gamma globulin.

A fortunate, if somewhat heartless, aspect of this story is that afflicted foals die off early and do not enter the breeding ranks to perpetuate their defects. The bacteria, then, control the appearance and incidence of such defects in foals by killing off the affected individuals.

This leads to a consideration of routine antibiotic administration to the newborn foal. This has become a common practise in many areas, the rationale being to give antibiotics before the bacteria arrive. The practise may be seriously questioned, however. If one is to operate on this basis, the foal should receive antibiotics regularly for at least two to three months after birth. A single "shot" shortly after birth will protect the foal for three or four days, the long acting preparations somewhat longer. However, the bacteria may develop resistance to the antibiotic. If infected later, then, with the resistant bacteria, the antibiotic will not be effective, and the foal will either die or its joints will be totally destroyed. Without belaboring the point, the best approach is adequate space, scrupulous sanitation, and careful, daily examination of every foal. Antibiotics are marvelous, but the careful eye of the good horseman is essential.

Foals infected with the rhinopneumonitis virus may be born at term. It is immediately apparent that something is gravely wrong. The affected individual shows severe respiratory distress: difficult, gasping breathing and bluish or gray-white mucous membranes. The lungs are severely damaged by the virus. While vigorous attempts have been made to treat such foals, it is true that most, if not all, will die within 24 to 48 hours. The lung damage is so extensive and comes at such a critical time, the transition from intra- to extrauterine life, that no amount or type of treatment can be successful.

The next area to be considered is an emotionally difficult one:—foals born with structural, *anatomical defects*. Oversimplifying enormously these defects fall into two categories: congenital—"accidental" improper formation of one or more parts, and hereditary—nonaccidental, gene-controlled improper formation of one or more parts. It is not always easy to differentiate between congenital and genetic. Fortunately, the incidence of such defects is not high in horses, but one must be prepared for them and be ready to bite the bullet when they appear.

Entropion is quite common in foals and may well be hereditary. Either the upper or lower eyelid (usually the lower) is turned in against the eyeball and causes irritation and inflammation of the eye. Conservative treatment (ointments and averting the eyelid several times a day) may be tried. Surgical correction, however, is easier, quicker and generally successful.

Contracted limbs, either the forelimbs (usually), rearlimbs or both are not uncommon. This condition has been described in *The Lame Horse*, and the reader is referred to that book for details. Although the evidence is incomplete, it appears that these contractures can be either congenital or hereditary. Some foals born with moderate or mild flexion contractures "walk out of" the contracture in a day or two. These are physiological contractures as a result of a crowding of the foal in the uterus during the latter part of pregnancy. Foals that do not walk out of the problem in a day or two have pathological contracture, and they should be examined by the veterinarian. The first objective is not to determine *how* to straighten the

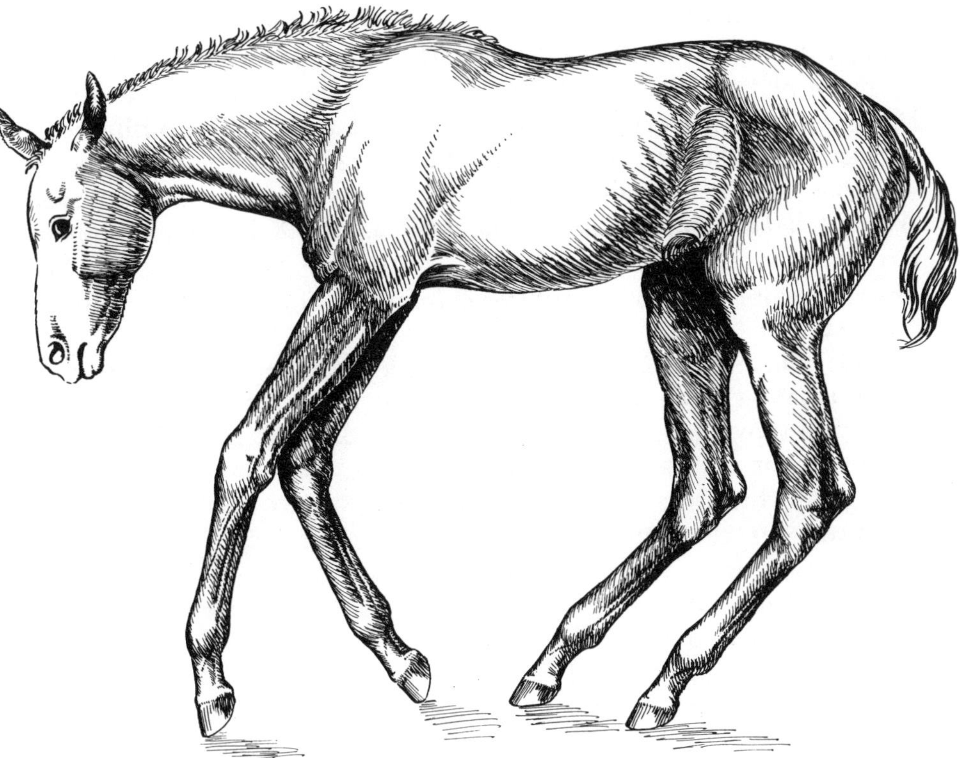

Fig. 19 Newborn foal with contracted forelimbs. The foal is unable to straighten the forelimbs and is camped under with the rearlegs to support itself.

legs but *if* they should be straightened. It is true that many of these contractures are the result of malformed bones and, if the contractures are straightened by casting or some other means, the animal will simply do it all over again when it becomes a yearling. The veterinarian and owner, together, must decide if the difficulty, expense and guarded prognosis justify an attempt to correct the problem. In the long run many of these foals must be destroyed.

Some foals seem to have just the opposite problem. The fetlocks, particularly of the rear legs, rest on the ground, and there seems to be too little action of the flexor muscles rather than too much as in the contracted foal. The cause of this condition is not known, but the majority of the affected foals develop muscle tone in a few days, and the fetlock moves up to normal position. Protect the fetlock for a few days with bandages, and the condition generally corrects itself.

Limb malformations, other than the above, are seen with some frequency and are probably hereditary in most cases. The commonest is

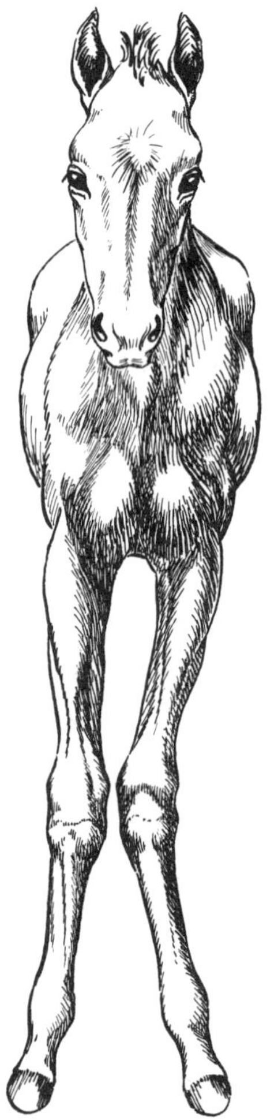

Fig. 20   A newborn foal with knock-knees as the result of improper development of the bones in or around the carpus.

so-called *knock-knee* affecting one or both front legs. The cause is delay in the development or frank hypoplasia of the small bones on the outside of the carpus. If delayed development, the bones may "catch up," and the leg straighten out. More commonly hypoplasia is the problem, and the legs cannot straighten on their own. Here is where the bullet-biting comes in. If after a reasonable period, two to three weeks probably, the foal is not improving on its own or is getting worse, the decision to put the foal down or resort to surgery must be made. It is certainly true that the surgical procedure (in one of its several forms) will straighten many of these legs. Surgery does not, however, correct the basic defect but, rather, creates another defect which counteracts the first one, so that the leg *looks* normal even though it is not normal and never will be. Will such a horse stand up under hard work? That question has never been answered by the advocates of surgery.

A variety of malformations can affect the head. Most of them are obvious, quickly lethal and need not be considered further. Occasionally a foal is born with *improperly developed eyes,* usually hypoplasia. The eyes are smaller than normal and completely disorganized. The foal is permanently blind and there is nothing to be done about it.

Cleft palate is seen infrequently and may be suspected when milk runs out of the nose of the nursing foal. This condition is probably hereditary and, though correctable by surgery in some cases, I doubt that they should be corrected.

Hernias are a common problem, and most of them seem to be hereditary. A hernia is a protrusion of something, usually a piece of intestine, through an abnormal opening or an opening which is normal except too large. The common sites are the umbilicus (normal but too large), the inguinal-scrotal area (normal but too large) and along the lower, ventral midline of the belly (abnormal opening).

The *umbilical hernia* is a failure of the normal opening through which the umbilical cord passed to close, allowing a loop of intestine or a lump of fat to bulge through the opening beneath the skin. Most of these hernias close without incident by one year of age. If not closed by then, they are readily repaired surgically.

Ventral hernia is failure of the belly wall to close at some point other than the umbilicus. Since, during early fetal life, the abdomen is normally wide open, it is perhaps not surprising that such a failure of closure can occur. Most of these hernias do not close spontaneously and must be repaired surgically.

Inguinal-scrotal hernias are protrusions through a too-large inguinal canal. The canal is the normal opening, one on each side of course, which allows the blood vessels and sperm-carrying duct (the ductus deferens) to pass from inside the abdomen to the testis. If this canal is too large, a loop of small intestine may protrude into the canal (inguinal hernia) or all the way into the scrotum (scrotal hernia). These hernias are dangerous since the loop of bowel may become entrapped, and its blood supply shut off, with fatal colic the end result. This area should always be carefully checked in any male horse with colic. Surgical repair is the only recourse once herniation occurs although the testis must usually be removed as well. That is just as well and take out the other testis as well because the condition is hereditary.

Atresia ani or *coli* is failure of development of the anus, rectum or higher segments of the large intestine. The foal is unable to defecate, needless to say, since it has no opening. Surgical repair is rarely successful and, since the condition is probably hereditary, that is just as well.

Leaving defects we come to the common problem of *meconium impaction.* Meconium is the waxy, semisolid material which accumulates in the lumen of the foal's intestinal tract during fetal life. It is a mixture of dead, sloughed epithelial cells (they die and slough off normally and are replaced), mucus, and amniotic fluid swallowed by the foal. As a rule this meconium is quickly passed soon after the foal nurses for the first time, activating the oral-anal reflex. If the meconium is not passed, the foal will show straining and colicky signs. The meconium may be removed by enema, the administration of fluids per rectum stimulating normal gut motility. This "sluggishness" of the intestine is peculiar to foals and may be related to the delayed coordination of gut movement which we discussed earlier with the premature foal. The maturation of the muscular and motor activity of the intestine is a real problem and mystery in the foal and needs study.

What enema and how? This job should be done by or under the guidance of a veterinarian. Only soft rubber tubes should be employed and abundant amounts of soapy water or a liquid surface tension reducing agent (detergent). Give a little, wait a little, give a little. Be patient and the meconium will begin to move eventually. Never use hard rubber tubes, human enema equipment, dose syringes and such. The rectum is easily torn by such devices, and too many foals have already died from lacerated rectums and subsequent peritonitis. Take it easy and get veterinary help if you've never done it before.

Rupture of the urinary bladder is another neonatal event peculiar to the foal. It occurs during the course of delivery, is most frequent in males, and afflicts about 0.1% of the foals born each year. The bladder of the foal may be full of urine when delivery begins. The urachus which carried urine from the bladder of the foal to the allantoic cavity is functionally closed at the time of birth. The penis of the male is compressed and shut down in the confines of the mare's bony pelvis during delivery. The pressure exerted on the foal's belly as it passes through the mare's pelvis causes rupture of the full bladder because urine cannot escape through either urachus or penis.

The clinical signs, of immediate interest, include depression and failure to nurse. The abdomen gradually becomes distended. The veterinarian can ballot (tap and listen) to the abdomen and hear the urine sloshing back and forth. He may confirm this by tapping the belly with a needle and smelling the fluid which is drawn off. This may not sound too nice, but years ago physicians diagnosed diabetes by tasting the urine. If it was sweet, sugar was present and that meant diabetes. The sophisticated laboratory can hardly do better.

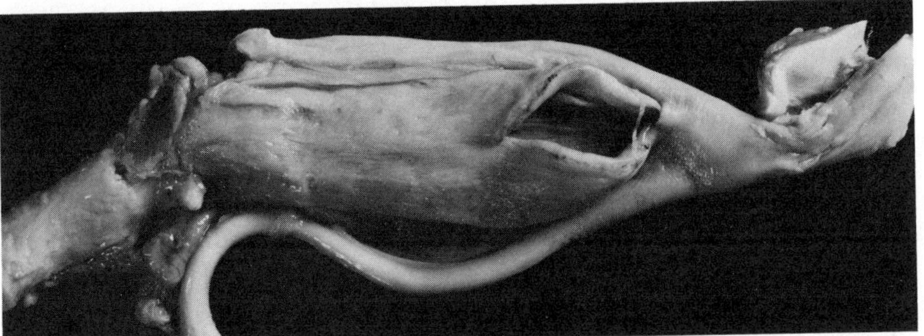

Fig. 21   Photograph of a ruptured urinary bladder.

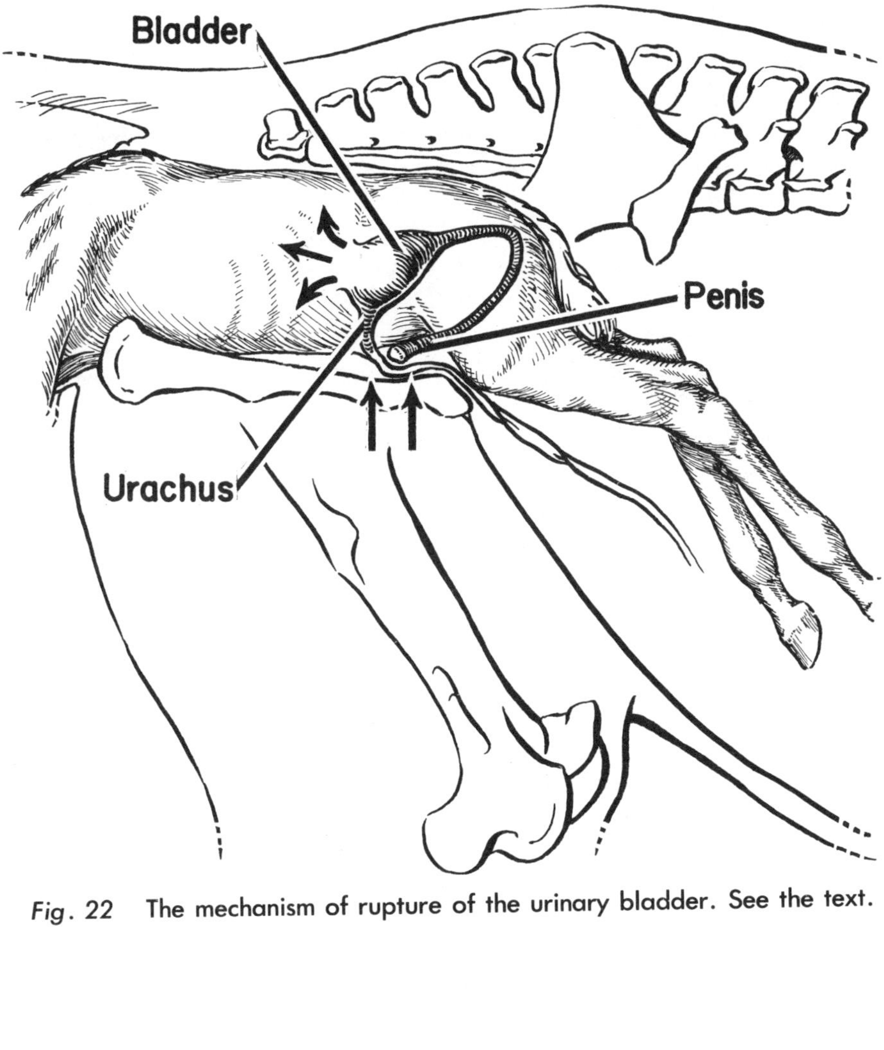

Fig. 22   The mechanism of rupture of the urinary bladder. See the text.

Once rupture has been diagnosed surgery is the only and best answer. The abdomen is opened, the tear sewn up and the urine removed. The foal usually recovers without difficulty.

"The foal is depressed." I've been saying that over and over again. Now it must be said about yet another condition: *hemolytic disease of the newborn.*

Depression and failure to nurse are the first signs of almost everything that goes wrong with the very young foal, and, obviously, can mean many different things. The veterinarian should be called immediately to examine the foal and determine the diagnosis. The foal should not be given a shot of pen-strep or something else and then "wait and see" attitude taken. The wait may be too long. Foals die of ruptured bladders, and hemolytic disease and bacterial infections.

Hemolytic disease is similar to though not identical with rH factor disease of the human infant. In simplest terms, the foal has a blood type different from that of the mare. Some of the foal's red blood cells (which carry the "type" or antigen) leak into the blood stream of the mare through the placenta. Since the foal's red blood cells are "foreign" to the mare, her immune system makes antibodies against the foal's red blood cells. If the mare's antibodies encounter the foal's red blood cells, the antibody will break up and agglutinate (clump) those cells. It is fortunate that antibody produced by the mare cannot pass through the placenta into the foal while it is still in the uterus. In the human, on the other hand, antibody can cross the placenta, and rH disease can develop in the infant before birth. After the foal is born it nurses the mare, taking in those anti-red cell antibodies with the first, colostral milk. Colostrum is very rich in antibody of all sorts, most of them beneficial, providing protection against infection during the first days and weeks of life. The colostral antibody can be absorbed through the wall of the foal's intestine for the first 48 hours after birth. After that, the wall "closes," and antibodies can no longer be absorbed from the gut into the foal's bloodstream. Obviously, if the mare has made antibody against the foal's red blood cells, this antibody, taken in with the colostrum, will be absorbed into the blood stream. Once there, it causes the foal's red blood cells to break down and/or agglutinate. The sudden loss, and destruction, of red cells causes acute, severe anemia. The foal stops nursing, and becomes weak and depressed. The mucous membranes will be very pale and may have a yellowish, jade green tinge. Laboratory examination will confirm the diagnosis. The foal should be muzzled immediately, so that no more antibodies are ingested. Blood transfusions may be necessary and, obviously, the blood should not come from the mother! In fact, it may be difficult to find a suitable donor horse, particularly if repeated transfusions are necessary. The foal should be given antibiotics (this is one time, anyway!)

to, in part, replace the absence of adequate colostral antibodies. The foal can be bottle-fed, and the mare milked out until 48 hours when the foal can be allowed to nurse again. Often it is more satisfactory to find a nurse mare, if available.

The most satisfactory approach to this problem is prevention. There are a number of strategies, of varying degrees of complexity, for accomplishing this. The simplest would seem to be taking some drops of the foal's blood, directly from the umbilical stump, mixing that blood with colostrum and observing the reaction. If the red cells are clumped by the colostrum, the foal should be muzzled and not allowed to nurse until the mare has been milked out for 48 hours. The foal will not ingest antibody and hemolytic disease will not occur. A veterinarian should be consulted and a program set up. Once a mare has been shown to react with her foal's red cells, one may assume that she will do it year after year (particularly, of course, if bred to the same or a related stallion).

For some years, a peculiar condition of the very young foal has been described in England and Ireland by the name *barker-wanderer-dummy*. Although these particular terms are not much used in the United States, we do have essentially the same condition or conditions. There is still considerable difference of opinion about this problem, and what I shall say is my opinion, as I see it.

The barker is a foal, usually only a few hours old, that suddenly begins to make desperate breathing movements accompanied by a gasping for air that sounds like a dog barking, and, hence, the name. Many of these foals show no other clinical signs and quickly die unless treated. Some foals recover from the gasping attacks without, or more often with, treatment and appear completely normal thereafter. Others may appear to recover from the acute attack only to become wanderers, walking aimlessly and almost continuously around the confines of stall or paddock. They appear stupid and even blind, but the eyes are normal. One grim example of such a foal was the offspring of a blind mare. The foal wore a bell, as is common practise with a blind mare. The foal wandered night and day, the bell ringing continuously. He was an utter dunce, and the poor mare was close to a nervous breakdown. This foal, as most of them, was put down. An occasional animal appears to recover from this stage. It is true, however, from the experience of a number of trainers, that individuals with this wanderer history are virtually untrainable as yearlings and two year olds. They simply do not have enough brain power to figure out what the trainer is trying to get them to do, even for racing.

As noted, the cause of this condition, or series of conditions, is in dispute. My experience has been that foals showing barking signs and dying have either a severe septicemia (generalized bacterial infection) with marked involvement of the lungs, or they have a severe disease restricted to the lungs alone. In either case, the lung problem leads to deficient oxygen exchange, air hunger, and the gasping clinical signs. Oxygen deficiency, particularly in early life when the brain is developing, can cause irreparable damage to the cerebrum. The clinical signs of wanderer and dummy are those of cerebral damage.

That's all fair enough, but what causes the septicemia and/or pneumonia? The septicemia can be caused by shigella, streptococcus, *E. coli* and probably some others. Any one of these bugs can also cause pneumonia alone. Often, by the time such a foal comes to postmortem, however, it has been so heavily treated with antibiotics that we are unable to grow the causative organisms. Microscopic sections show bacteria in the lungs, but they cannot be identified by this means. Obviously, the infection is contracted before, during or immediately after birth since the clinical signs appear as early as a few hours after birth.

While on the subject of pneumonia, it is apropos to discuss a unique pneumonia of foals, *adenoviral pneumonia*, that has recently been defined. The virus attacks, primarily, Arabian foals of a particular genetic line. A few cases have been seen in Thoroughbreds.

The adenovirus afflicts the specific Arabians because they are genetically deficient in the immunoglobulins which form antibodies as discussed earlier. The virus is breathed in and sets up infection in the lungs. The foal may die of the viral infection or become secondarily infected with the bacterium *Corynebacterium equi*.

It is an interesting fact that the same Arabian blood lines susceptible to the adenovirus are the ones which are afflicted with cerebellar hypoplasia. That will be discussed in a later chapter. A reasonable, though unproven, relationship may be the following: The adenovirus invades the pregnant mare, travels to the uterus in her bloodstream and sets up an infection in the developing brain of the fetus. By the time the foal is born the infection has run its course and disappeared but the cerebellum has been irreparably damaged by the virus, and this damage, then, appears as hypoplasia. That's reasonable since the developing nerve cells have been destroyed and are not there to develop. While not demonstrated in foals, this mechanism has been shown to be operative in cats with a respiratory virus disease.

Corynebacterium equi is a saprophytic, soil-living bacterium which can do enormous damage to young foals, generally around the age of three to four months. *C. equi* is not a good pathogen as bacteria go and needs help in order to set up infection in the foal. It has already been noted that adenovirus is one of those helping hands. Any foal that has severe problems, particularly of the respiratory, digestive, or immune systems, is a candidate for *C. equi* infection. The weak, sick, and deficient, then, are the animals primarily at risk. The organism gains entry to the body through the air passages, but it may be taken in with food as well.

The clinical signs can vary. The susceptible foal exposed to a dusty paddock may receive such a large dose of bacteria that an acute, overwhelming pneumonia develops, the animal dying in a matter of hours. This form of the disease, while uncommon, is usually overlooked or misdiagnosed even at postmortem. Adenovirus and *C. equi* may strike almost simultaneously, producing an acute form of the disease. Careful laboratory work is required to sort them out.

The usual clinical picture is that of the foal that develops clear cut signs of pneumonia that do not respond to antibiotics within forty-eight to seventy-two hours. This resistance to antibiotics is quite characteristic of *C. equi* infection. The afflicted foal won't die and won't get well. It will just tool along, not growing, but wasting away, gradually becoming weaker. There are large abscesses in the lungs which are slow to heal. If forced to exercise, the foal will tire quickly, and one of the abscesses may break down and spread to the rest of the lung, causing a quickly fatal acute pneumonia.

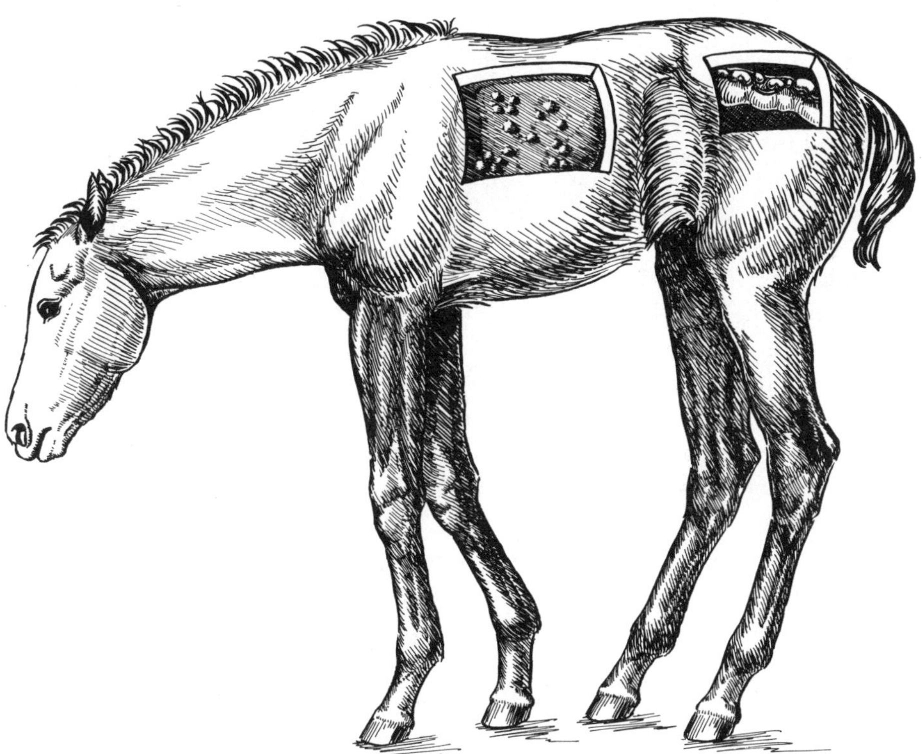

Fig. 23   Drawing indicating the sites of abscess formation (lung and gut), caused by *Corynebacterium equi* infection.

The intestinal tract may be involved alone (rarely) or together with the lungs. The signs described above are, then, accompanied by a persistent, intractable diarrhea which does not respond to routine therapy.

What does one do when this pattern of chronic, persistent infection of lung and gut is present? It is difficult. Prolonged antibiotic therapy (a month at least) is necessary and without guarantee of ultimate success. All efforts to produce a vaccine have failed (and if the immune system is defective that is perfectly reasonable. No vaccine can work if the body cannot respond to it).

Diarrhea is a common clinical sign in young foals that something is wrong but not, necessarily, what is wrong. That is important. Too often the horseman wants to treat the diarrhea with one of many products available, forgetting that the underlying disease, causing the diarrhea, is the important thing. Obviously kaolin and pectin aren't going to do a thing for abscessing *C. equi* infection of the gut. Diarrhea, then, is a clear warning to the owner to find out what is wrong!

One of the commoner causes of diarrhea in the foal is the animal's curiosity. The foal will pick up and eat all sorts of strange and wonderful things that do not agree with the intestine's idea of what should be inside it. The intestine's reaction to something which does not belong is to move faster and rush that obnoxious material to the outside. Brief bouts of soft manure caused by such curiosity eating are of no real concern.

Nine day scours is a most interesting condition. Often, when the mare is coming into heat for the first time after foaling, her foal will have diarrhea for a day or two. The foal rarely appears ill or goes off feed and, as a rule, recovers without complication. The cause of this condition is not known though several ideas have been put forth. The most reasonable explanation at the present time is that the scours are caused by a sudden change in the bacterial population in the lumen of the intestinal tract. The intestinal tract is normally inhabited by a variety of bacteria, fungi, and protozoa that do no harm and, by making certain nutrients available to the horse, actually do good. If a new population of any of these organisms suddenly develops in the gut around nine days (for reasons yet unknown), the gut will consider them strangers at first and try to get rid of them; hence, diarrhea.

Treatment is usually not necessary. I emphasize again, however, that diarrhea, even at nine days, is a sign that something is wrong. Something is in the gut that does not belong there. The animal should be checked to be sure that nothing is seriously wrong.

We have already noted that shigella, coli, and streptococci may, as they cause generalized disease (septicemia), cause diarrhea as well. A specific diarrhea-inducing organism of serious importance is salmonella. Two species, *Salmonella typhimurium* and *Salmonella enteriditis*, are commonly responsible for disease in horses. The first sign of infection is usually a severe diarrhea. The foal runs a high fever and goes off feed. The infection quickly spreads from foal to foal until all or nearly all are ill. The infection generally strikes when the foals are three to four months of age, but that is not invariable. The diarrhea is so severe and profuse that the animal quickly becomes dehydrated. That is, it loses so much fluid from the gut that it cannot be replaced as fast as it is being lost, and fluids are extracted from the body tissues. The foal is not nursing, and this adds to the fluid deficit problem. The treatment should be under a veterinarian's supervision. He will use antibiotics such as neomycin and chemotherapeutic agents such as furadantin and may have to supply fluids by stomach tube or vein in order to combat the dehydration.

With care and intensive nursing many foals will survive this infection. One must be on the lookout, however, for the occasional animal that seems to be recovering only to suddenly develop signs of joint infection and/or lameness. The salmonellae can escape from the gut and establish horrible infections in both joints and bones. These infections are difficult, if not impossible, to treat with any hope of a sound animal in the end. Fortunately, very few animals develop this problem. Thorough and early treatment must be used, trying to prevent the bacteria from escaping from the gut. If it does escape, and the antibiotics do not control, the horse could have a defective immune system, as discussed above.

Once salmonella infection has appeared on a farm, it is seeded there, and one can expect a new outbreak the following year. It may not, but the risk is always there. Faced with that unpleasant fact, the horseman may wish to consult his veterinarian about having a bacterin made to administer to each new crop of foals. There is no commercial bacterin available, so it must be made to order.

Salmonella can also infect older horses and, though this chapter is about foals, the problem of infection of older horses will be discussed here. The normal adult horse is quite resistant to salmonella in contrast to the foal. Whenever an older horse is under severe stress, however, and salmonella is around, infection can occur. The reasons are rather complex and not all that clear. The clinical signs, however, are essentially identical to those in the foal. As a rule, only one horse is involved, and the disease does not spread to normal, unstressed horses. If there are other animals under stress, however, the infection can spread.

In both foals and older horses, *supportive therapy* is as important as antibiotics in the treatment of salmonellosis as well as many other conditions. In fact, such therapy is important enough to warrant a digression.

It is completely true that for many diseases, in all species, there are no specific treatments available. Rather than specific treatment, however, therapy is directed to supporting and assisting the animal body as it mobilizes its own defenses against the attack of outside agents. The fluid therapy mentioned is an example. Not only must the specific cause be treated, but the resulting dehydration as well. Often, in fact, the effects of the disease are treated only because the cause is not known. While the white blood cells and antibodies are trying to deal with the invader, fluids that are being lost in the battle are being provided as part of the treatment. Help is given wherever possible, but the main battle is being fought by the animal itself. It is extremely important that the animal's defenses not be hindered by the treatment, however. This is one of the problems of modern medicine. There are so many powerful drugs available that there is a tendency to overdo, at unnecessary expense, even to the point of being counterproductive. Evidence is slowly accumulating that many drugs that are used freely have undesirable side effects.

Every so often, for example, one hears of the sudden death of a horse on a race track following the use of certain drugs or vitamins. The cause of death is usually anaphylactic shock. This is an unusual or exaggerated reaction of the animal to a foreign protein. For example, if a small quantity of egg albumin is injected beneath the horse's skin once and then again two weeks later, anaphylactic shock occurs. The horse does not react to the first injection, but it does form antibodies which will combine with the egg white of the second injection and cause a severe and, perhaps fatal, reaction.

This may occur with substances other than animal protein; for example, certain drug products. In some instances, the reaction may come after one or more injections, while, in other cases, the horse may react the first time it receives the drug. In the latter case, it may be said that the animal is sensitive, inherently, to that drug. We don't really know what that means, but it is something to say and is not untrue.

Specifically, I have seen immediately fatal responses to the injection of various preparations of vitamins A, D, E. I don't know why some horses are sensitive to these preparations nor am I aware of any work attempting to demonstrate why some react the way they do. As in so many other things in horse medicine, we operate with insufficient knowledge. Again, there seems to be no readily available way to predict how a given animal will react. You give the shot and take your chances which is rather tough with a first class horse.

The proper question to ask then, is: why give the vitamins by injection in the first place? I am sure those who do it have many reasons, but it is true that vitamins can be taken orally, and do their work without the risk of fatal injection reactions. Too frequently, in this hurry-up world, we feel that short-cuts are justified or, even more foolishly, that something given through a needle is better than something given or taken in by natural routes.

The "jug" of fluids frequently given to race horses may be questioned on similar grounds. If the animal has an adequate diet and free access to all the water he wishes to drink, there seems little justification for intravenous administration of fluids. Many feel that this magic jug moves a horse up (improves his racing) legally (or, at least, undetectably), but has that idea ever been scrupulously tested? If the horse begins to lose condition, dry up and do poorly, he needs a rest and some decent grazing more than he does water and drugs into his vein. Russian roulette with a hypodermic needle is not good horse husbandry!

Nursing care requires some comment. The life or death of a sick animal is as much in the hands of the attendant as it is of the veterinarian. While the sick human receives both medical and nursing attention, careful diet, rest and kind words, too often the horse simply gets a few "shots," that are supposed to cure everything. The veterinarian can diagnose, administer appropriate medicines, or counsel that none are needed. It is up to the attendants, with the veterinarian's advice, to provide the essential nursing care: fresh water, bits of carrot, some fresh grass, a gentle caress, a kind word. (People talk to plants, don't they!) Too often when the veterinarian says nothing is needed but rest and time, the owner is not satisfied. Off he goes to the neighbor or to the drug store, and the poor brute is pumped full of some tonic recommended by a feed store clerk or pharmacist who has never been within twenty feet of a horse. Medicine is not magic and often medical science is as much intelligent guesswork as hard fact. But, if in trouble, I should rather have intelligent guesswork than dumb guesswork!

5
RESPIRATORY DISEASE

With this chapter, the sequential, chronological approach which has been followed so far will be abandoned. From here on, problems will be discussed in terms of specific organs and tissues. Many of these things involve horses of any age, but specific age relationships will be noted where appropriate.

VIRAL RESPIRATORY DISEASE—INFLUENZA

There are four viruses known to cause respiratory infection in horses: rhinopneumonitis, adenovirus, influenza I and influenza II. The first two have been discussed and influenza remains.

At present, there are two influenza viruses known in the United States. There may be others but we do not know of them so far. Influenza typically infects a number of horses at the same or nearly the same time. Both influenza I and II have been in this country for some time, and most older horses have experienced the disease and are resistant to reinfection. The disease may be expected, then, primarily in young horses. If a new mutant of the virus appears (which is likely sooner or later), horses of all ages will be affected.

Infected horses run a fever, go off feed and will have a variably copious nasal discharge. Often there will be a dry cough (not seen with rhinopneumonitis infection). The virus invades the lining cells of the nose, trachea and lungs causing death of the cells and acute inflammation. There is no specific antibiotic or chemical which will kill influenza virus in the animal. One must, then, provide supportive treatment and wait for

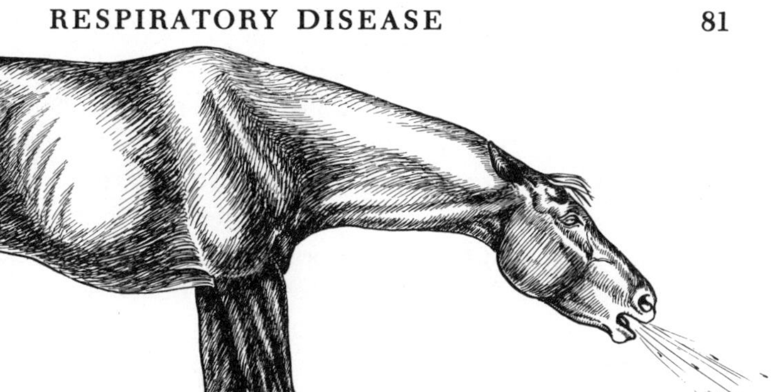

Fig. 24 Horse with a cough.

the animal's defenses to overcome the viral assault. While many things can and have been done, the best regimen (for this and any other respiratory disease) would seem to be the use of a sulfa drug and complete stall rest. The sulfa is to protect the horse from invasion by streptococci while rest allows the natural defenses to work at their best. Effective vaccines are available, but they are used to prevent and not to treat the disease once established.

The evidence indicates that administration of influenza and rhino-pneumonitis vaccines to young horses before they go into training significantly reduces the incidence of respiratory infection. It is important to administer the vaccines *before* heavy work begins because it is clear that the animal may have an adverse reaction to the vaccine once work is underway. There is no reaction to speak of in the non-working horse.

It is important to realize, and frequently forgotten, that the damage done by the influenza virus (or any other virus, for that matter) may take a considerable time to heal. In the case of influenza II, for example, it is known that damage is still present, not yet healed, as long as three weeks after all clinical signs of illness have disappeared. That fact leads to the following important narrative:

PLEURITIS

A horse on the racetrack develops an upper respiratory infection with fever and a watery nasal discharge. He is left in the stall, treated one way or another, and seems to be completely recovered and back to normal in five or six days. He is put back to work and, in a few days, is sick again with a high fever and a nasty, purulent nasal discharge. The horse was put back to work before the ulcers in the lining of the nose caused by virus had healed. The ubiquitous streptococcus moved into the damaged areas and set up a secondary, purulent infection. The horse is treated again and may be recovering nicely in a week or so. He is put back to work yet again or shipped to another area, often back to the farm because training has been set back. In a short time the animal is suddenly in dire straights. There is a high, fluctuating fever and difficult, labored breathing. The veterinarian listens to the chest and percusses it (tapping and listening for the sound of fluid) and says that the horse has pleuritis. Pleuritis (often called pleurisy) is a severe inflammation and infection of the lining of the chest cavity with the spilling of large quantities of fluid, pus, and fibrin (the stuff of blood clots) into the cavity. Heroic treatment with antibiotics together with drainage of fluid from the chest is now necessary. A few afflicted horses will recover, particularly if the treatment is started early. Many never recover and a few recover only to become chronic invalids.

What happened, bad luck? Not likely. During the course of that second, bacterial respiratory infection, some of the infectious material went down into the lung instead of out the nose. It set up a single abscess in the right lung. When the horse was worked or shipped (stressed, in other words), this abscess began to leak streptococci into the chest cavity, and the pleuritis was off and running. Unfortunately, the first signs of developing pleuritis may be quite subtle, and the disease can be well-advanced before it is correctly diagnosed.

Even if one can save the horse, and it's not easy, the expense of the antibiotics, nursing care, and so on, is horrendous. Prevention is the answer. Any horse that is working should have a minimum of three and preferably four weeks of rest following recovery from even an apparently mild respiratory infection. Note, particularly, that the animal should rest *where it is* and not be shipped. The trainer may complain that such a rest is impossible, and it probably is for the training schedule. It's either rest or the possibility of a dead horse.

Although it sounds terribly old-fashioned, I have seen several cases of pleuritis saved because of first class nursing care and a mustard plaster. While pouring in the antibiotics, keep the animal warm and quiet, offer fresh water frequently, tempt with green grass or carrots, and apply a mustard plaster over the chest (perhaps the electric blanket would work, too). Heat applied to the outside of the chest will increase the flow of blood within the chest, and that increased flow might be the edge you need to save the horse.

ROARING

So-called wind problems of one sort or another are legion in horses. They are of obvious importance because a horse cannot work efficiently if the flow of air in and out of the lungs is obstructed. The classical wind problem is roaring. This is a paralysis of the muscles on one side of the larynx (usually) which allows the vocal fold to hang loosely in the airway, flopping about and interfering with the normal flow of air. The loose vocal fold causes the sound which gives the condition its name. The paralysis is the result of damage to the nerve (left recurrent nerve) which supplies the muscles of the left side of the larynx. The cause of that damage is still in dispute but clearly associated with large horses with long necks. Man has selected for larger horses and long necks (compare the Thoroughbred

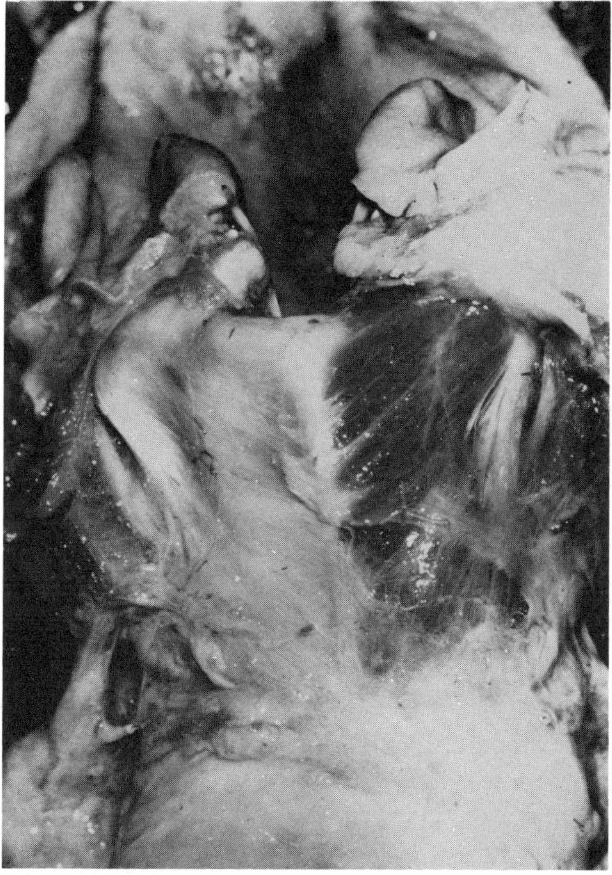

Fig. 25 Photograph of the larynx of a horse that was a roarer. The normal muscle is to the right and dark in color while the atrophied muscle to the left is light.

with the parent stock Arabian type). While this greater size is an advantage to man in that the horse can run faster and jump better, it does predispose the horse to roaring and wobbles (see *The Lame Horse* pp. 220-223 for discussion of wobbles).

The veterinarian can confirm the diagnosis of roaring by looking at the larynx through a lighted tube called a rhinolaryngoscope and seeing the paralyzed vocal fold. A relatively simple operation corrects the problem in many horses. The sac next to the vocal fold is stripped out. As the area heals, the vocal fold is stuck and held against the wall of the larynx, so that it no longer obstructs the airway. It may not work the first time, necessitating a second operation. A more complicated procedure is being used by some surgeons, involving replacement of the lost, paralyzed muscle with a plastic strap to hold the vocal fold to the side of the larynx. This is a sound theoretical approach to the problem, but its long range practicability has yet to be determined.

PROBLEMS IN THE PHARYNX

Some horses make noises and have air problems without paralysis of the larynx. The cause in many of these cases is not known and/or subject to dispute. I'll tell you what I know and think. Not everyone agrees with me, and you should know that, too!

A definite cause of airway obstruction, however, is the presence of loose, floppy folds of the wall of the pharynx. They can obstruct the flow of air and can be seen with the rhinolaryngoscope. Surgical removal is usually successful. The cause is not known, but most cases have been in Standardbred horses, suggesting a hereditary basis.

The *soft palate* may obstruct the airway. There are two stated causes only one of which I believe. "Too long" soft palate is often described. I have never seen one. Partial or complete paralysis of the muscles of the soft palate seems quite clear although I have had no opportunity to study one at postmortem. The surgeons remove a portion of the soft palate, clearing the airway despite the paralysis and, thus, the pathologist doesn't see them.

So-called *chronic pharyngitis* is often cited as a cause of wind problems and coughing. Mucus, pus, and reddening of the wall of the pharynx are seen with the lighted "scope." I believe this material has come up into the pharynx from the bronchi and trachea, and the basic problem, then, is chronic bronchitis-tracheitis and not pharyngitis at all. I have never seen a *bona fide* case of pharyngitis at postmortem while chronic bronchitis is often seen. Since the treatment for pharyngitis and bronchitis is essentially the same, it's not easy to decide what has been cured, if and when it is cured. The whole story is yet to be told.

CHRONIC COUGH

To my knowledge there are two major causes of chronic coughing in horses. The first is the exposure of the animal to allergens which are often present in dusty bedding and/or forage. As in humans, some horses will be sensitive and react to these allergens (like hay fever) while others do not. The allergen calls forth an antibody, and the combination of allergen and antibody induces an inflammatory reaction, primarily in the smaller air passages of the lung (the bronchioles). The natural reaction of the air passages to the presence of irritants and/or inflammation is the initiation of the cough reflex. The object of the coughing is to rid the air passage of the irritant substances and products of the inflammatory reaction. If, however, the inflammation persists long enough or recurs frequently enough, permanent damage is done to the muscle tissue surrounding the bronchioles. As a result the lung is unable to clear air normally, and the condition known as *heaves* develops. This type of cough, then, can be called allergic bronchitis or bronchiolitis, and it can occur and recur over and over again until, eventually, permanent damage is done.

Heaves is simply the end stage of bronchitis and is characterized clinically by loss of weight, coughing, and marked difficulty in expelling air from the lungs. The marked effort of the abdominal muscles, attempting to help the lungs expel air, produces a line in the muscles of the flank, behind the last rib, known as the "heave line."

There are several approaches to this problem. First, and obviously, one must try to reduce the exposure of the susceptible horse to allergens. This includes wetting the hay before feeding, feeding pellets, avoiding straw or other dusty bedding, and avoiding dry, dusty paddocks, or show rings. The ventilation of the barn must be closely checked. If the rate of air flow is too slow, allergens can accumulate in the humid, stagnant air. While gales of wind are not wanted, every effort should be made to avoid stagnant air. Steroids and antibiotics can be administered to afflicted horses for a week or so in order to alleviate the clinical signs. This is not a cure, however. The condition will recur if allergens are not controlled. Sensitivity testing, as done with humans, has not been done to any great extent with the horse but may offer another tool (desensitization) once the necessary research has been done.

The second cause of chronic coughing *may* be infection of the air passages by specific viruses. ("may" because there has been very little work to support or deny the idea). If viral irritation and damage is followed by secondary bacterial infection, or the linings of the air passages are rendered sensitive to allergens because of the damage, a chronic disease state is set in train. The prevention and treatment, happily, is essentially the same as given above: basically, to avoid exposure to humid, stagnant air loaded with allergens, viruses and bacteria. Chronic coughing is primarily a disease of stabled horses and thereby hangs the tale!

BLEEDER

Epistaxis, bleeding from the nose, is not an uncommon problem of working horses, particularly racing horses. There are several causes to be considered.

The first is infection in the guttural pouches, either one or, less commonly, both. This infection occurs sporadically and is distinctly life-endangering as we shall see. First of all, what is a guttural pouch and what does it do? It is a sac-like outpouching of the eustachian tube. We all have eustachian tubes running from the pharynx to the cavity of the

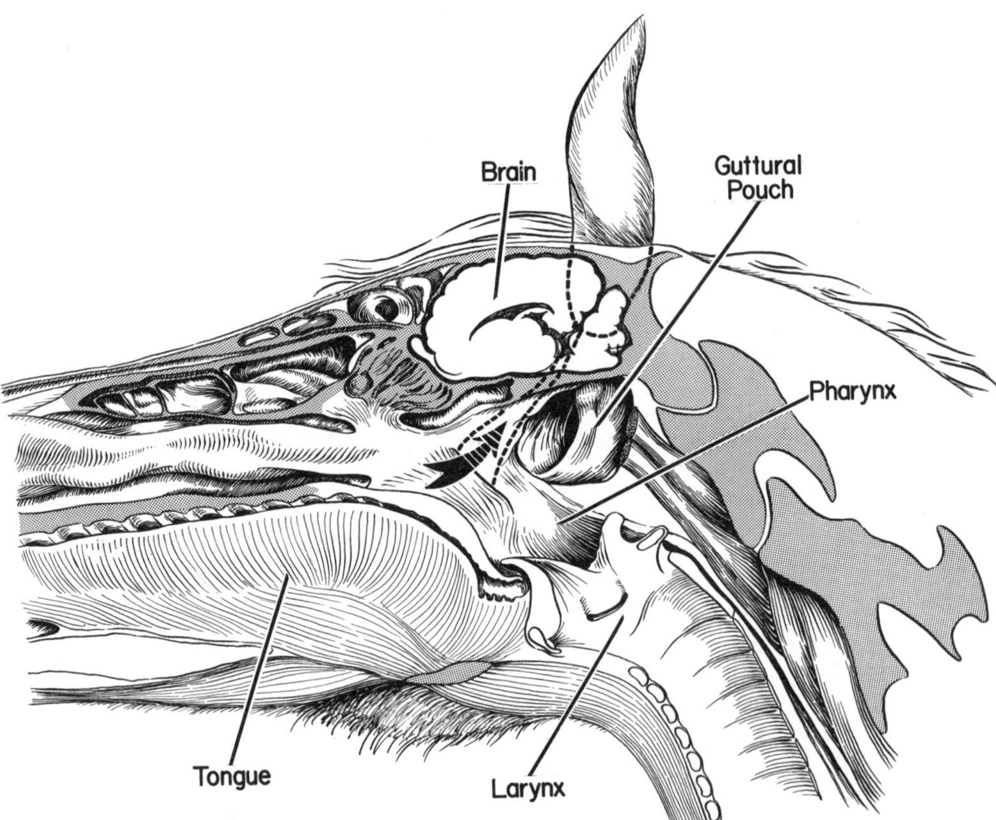

Fig. 26　Split section of a horse's head showing the location of the guttural pouch on one side. The arrow indicates the movement of air into the pouch from the pharynx.

middle ear. The movement of air through these tubes keeps the pressure within the middle ear the same as in the pharynx. Air moving through that tube is what "opens" ears when yawning or swallowing in an airplane. It is the air not moving, causing a pressure difference between ear and throat, that causes the full feeling in the ear. In the horse and his relatives, the rhinocerous and the tapir (did you know that?), a large pouch is developed as part of this tube. There has been very little work on the function of these pouches. It is possible, on theoretical grounds, that the guttural pouches serve as pressure balancing devices, storing air in the pouches when pressure in the pharnx in high and releasing it again into the pharynx when pharyngeal pressure drops. Such a drop in pressure could allow the pharynx to collapse upon itself, shutting off or, at least, reducing the flow of air. Braving the dangers of teleological thinking, this pressure balancing mechanism may have developed because the horse moves such large volumes of air with his large chest and lungs. The mechanism, then, would be particularly important during exercise when the amount of air being moved through the passages approaches a maximum.

The common infection in the guttural pouch is related to a fungus (*Aspergillus*) which localizes in the upper part of the pouch where air entering the pouch strikes the lining (an impingement point). Although unproven, it might be suggested that a virus does the initial damage allowing the fungus to set up a secondary infection. Unfortunately, there are a number of important structures in the area where the fungus localizes.

Specifically, nerves supplying the soft palate pass through this area (and paralysis of the soft palate is seen in some cases of guttural pouch infection) as does the internal carotid artery which supplies blood to the brain. The fungus has an unfortunate affinity for blood vessels and sooner or later grows into the wall of the internal cartoid artery. Blood, then, leaks or flows from the damaged artery into the guttural pouch. When the horse lowers its head to eat, for example, the blood runs out of the pouch and gushes from the nose. The bleeding can be so extensive and severe that the horse goes into shock and dies. Eventually, most horses so affected do just that. The veterinarian can confirm the diagnosis by examining the pouch with the scope. Treatment, at present, is not satisfactory. I can only suggest that the veterinarian try whatever he can think of and let us all know if it works!

The commonest type of bleeding, seen in racing horses, is not so fatal and extensive, or rarely so. The typical story is that the horse leaves the gate fast, bobbles at the ⅛ pole, finishes the race, usually back in the pack, returns to the paddock, coughs, and, finally, bleeds from the nose. This bleeding is from the lung in virtually all, if not all, cases.

The reasoning, briefly, is as follows, If, for any reason, a horse holds its breath or breathes irregularly, air will not move smoothly through the air passages and may remain trapped for a time in the lung. This entrapped air distends the air spaces, and those distended air spaces slow the flow of venous blood out of the lungs. The back pressure thus developed in the veins results in poor oxygenation of the walls of the veins with damage to the walls the inevitable result. Blood moves through the damaged walls into the air spaces and is quickly carried up the bronchi and trachea (about five minutes more or less from lung to throat and nose). The blood travels up the air passages in the blanket of mucus normally lining these passages, and this mucus is propelled toward the throat by tiny cilia on the surface of the air passage lining cells.

The cough, after the race, is induced by the blood entering the pharynx. Why the bobble at the ⅛ pole? It seems to be true that many horses will hold their breath when they leave the starting gate as an "aid" to moving faster. Human athletes do this as well, deliberately, for short distance swimming and running races. One moves faster for short distances by holding one's breath. Interestingly, these human sprinters often bleed after a race, too! At the ⅛ pole (or thereabouts) the horse must begin to breath and to synchronize that breathing with the gait. He bobbles, or seems to, then, as he shifts gait in order to synchronize his breathing.

While a characteristic story, this is not the only way that bleeding into the lungs can be induced. The unfit and/or exhausted horse, as at the end of grueling cross country race, may breath irregularly, incompletely emptying the lungs because of the gasping, irregular breathing pattern. Also, though there is not direct evidence as yet, atrial fibrillation may cause backing up of blood in the lung and predispose the animal to bleeding.

Once the damage has been done to the veins in the lung, scar tissue will develop in the damaged vessels and, since scar tissue is never as strong as normal tissue, the tendency to repeated damage and repeated bleeding is established. In fact, repeated damage to the veins may reach such proportions that even normal breathing during light work or racing may cause rupture and bleeding. It has been noted, in the past, that this type of bleeding seems to have a hereditary tendency, perhaps because certain lines of horses tend to hold their breath or to tire for reasons quite unrelated to the lungs.

There have been many forms of treatment for bleeders. Since there have been no controlled experiments no one can say just what does and does not work. True prevention would seem to lie in training the horse gradually up to the work he must do, not asking more than possible, stopping when fatigued and instructing jockeys not to let the horse breath hold out of the gate. The latter might be accomplished by not going away quite so fast. Some ground will be lost, obviously, but I guess that's better than coming in last and bleeding all over the paddock.

Many people feel that there are bleeding points in the nose, throat (or somewhere!) which are responsible for bleeding. That may be true in isolated cases, but it does not appear to be a common cause of bleeding. All the evidence points to the lung as the major site of damage in the common racetrack bleeder.

STRANGLES

Strangles is one of the more important, but generally nonfatal, bacterial diseases of the horse. It is caused by a specific organism (*Streptococcus equi*). The horse acquires this disease by exposure to the nasal secretions and/or pus of another horse that has the disease. Buckets, rags, and even a person's hands contaminated by infected pus from a sick horse can serve as the source of infection as well. Four to five days after exposure the horse will show clinical signs. The animal will stop eating and drinking and may run a fever (102-106° F.). A copious nasal discharge often occurs.

The bacteria invade the lining of the throat and produce small abscesses. These abscesses break down and drain through the nose as well as moving to and infecting the lymph nodes around the throat area. These lymph nodes become inflammed and swell markedly. They are generally seen and felt in the throatlatch area and cause the horse considerable pain and discomfort.

Within ten days to two weeks after the onset of the infection, these abscessed lymph nodes will break through the skin and drain to the outside. Healing begins and the animal will be nearly immune to further infection—note that I said "nearly immune." If the horse is reexposed some time later, however, he may be reinfected, but this second attack is generally much milder and rarely progresses to the stage of frank abscessation and draining pus.

In general, when strangles is introduced to a herd, almost every susceptible animal will, sooner or later, show clinical signs of disease. In fact, once the disease has become established on a farm it may appear at any time in new horses brought to the farm and in each succeeding crop of foals.

This leads to a major point about disease control, strangles or any other infectious disease, on horse farms. While frequently difficult to accomplish, quarantine of all new arrivals on a farm should be practised. As a rule of thumb any new horse brought to the farm should be isolated from the "home" animals for a period of two to three weeks. While the incubation period for strangles is only one week, there are a number of other infectious diseases with considerably longer incubation periods.

In the wild state, the horse rambled over many miles of range and the concentration of infectious diseases, such as strangles, was always low. Sick individuals would drop out of the herd, automatically removing themselves as a source of contagion to other animals. Indeed, predators frequently served to remove the sick individual altogether. Man, however, for obvious reasons, bands horses together in small areas, concentrating both the horses and their diseases. Since we cannot duplicate the wild state, we must do the best we can with what we have. Quarantine is, therefore, one of the most important single tools available to the farm operator in the task of avoiding outbreaks of infectious diseases such as strangles.

What constitutes an effective quarantine? Obviously, two separate farms would be ideal but hardly practical for most operations. Under usual conditions there should be a separate paddock or small field with a barn—or, better yet, an open shed—which is a minimum of 100 yards from the nearest home horses. It has been shown that respiratory viruses cannot survive a trip of that distance without being dried out and killed.

Again, ideally, those people who care for quarantined animals should not come in contact with the home horses. If this is not possible, the caretakers should feed, clean, and otherwise care for the home horses first, moving to the quarantined animals only after all the work has been done with the home horses.

Why an open shed rather than a barn? Barns tend to accumulate things such as dried pus, contaminated feed sacks and so on. Barns tend to be damp with poor air circulation. The open shed is easily cleaned and the best disinfectants, fresh air and sunlight, are available in abundance.

As noted, once strangles is introduced, most horses will be infected. Most will recover. An occasional individual may develop so-called "bastard strangles" in which the disease spreads from the throat to other parts of the body. While it may spread anywhere there is a distinct tendency for an unsuspected abscess to develop in the lower part of the neck. This abscess may fill the space between the first two ribs and shut off the windpipe, resulting in suffocation.

Foals infected early in life may develop septicemia and die. In both the foal and the individual inadequate defense mechanisms rather than differences in the organism seem to be most the important cause of bastard strangles.

Some clinical observations suggest that improper treatment with penicillin may increase the incidence of bastard strangles. The penicillin kills many of the bacteria but, in so doing, may prevent the animal from developing adequate natural antibodies against the infection and, thereby, allow it to spread to other parts of the body. In general, it appears best to wait for the abscesses to drain before penicillin is administered.

There is evidence that many horses develop changes in the normal electrical activity of the heart during strangles infection. It would be desireable, then, to have the heart carefully checked before returning the animal to work.

Another untoward aftereffect of strangles infection may be the condition known as *purpura hemorrhagica*. In this severe and dangerous condition there is marked illness and depression with bleeding and accumulation of fluid beneath the skin and in the muscles. Purpura appears to be an allergic reaction provoked by the streptococcus. Mild cases of purpura usually recover easily, but the condition is dangerous and veterinary help should be quickly sought.

There is a bacterin for the prevention of strangles infection. It is rather a rough vaccine on the horse, however, and should be given only and strictly according to the recommendations of the manufacturer and the veterinarian. One cannot emphasize too strongly, however, that strict quarantine and stable hygiene are the best preventitives for strangles.

6

HEART

Any discussion of the myriad disorders, would-be disorders and may-be disorders of the horse's heart is fraught with severe difficulty. While I can tell you with some clarity about fatal disorders of the heart, nonfatal disorders, evaluated by clinical means, still remain a complex and confusing area.

CONGENITAL DEFECTS

While congenital defects of the heart do occur in horses, they seem to be much less common than in most other domestic animals. The reason would seem to be that those animals that have performed with some success as athletes are selected for breeding, and such success presupposes cardiovascular soundness. Dogs, cows, pigs, etc. are selected for reasons other than athletic ability, and congenital defects are more common than in the horse.

There is little merit to a recital of all the various things that can go awry during the embryological development of the heart. The most common defect is what is called an interventricular septal defect, a failure of the wall between the two ventricles of the heart to form completely. This allows blood from the two sides to mix. Since this mixing of blood is the basic functional problem in many congenital defects, it is worth considering in some detail. During fetal life, blood rich in oxygen flows into the fetus from the placenta by way of the umbilical veins, through the liver and into the right side (atrium) of the heart. Since the fetal lungs are not necessary to supply oxygen to the blood (and, obviously, cannot do so)

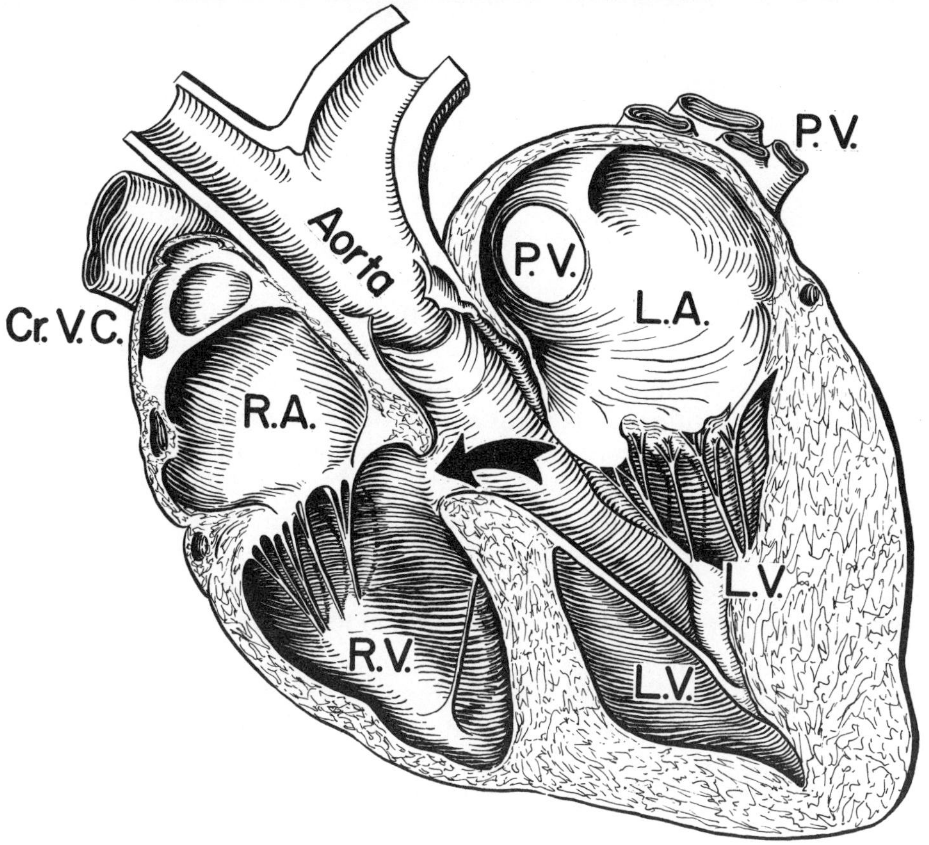

Fig. 27   Section of a horse's heart. The arrow indicates a defect in the septum between the two ventricles of the heart. Cr. V.C. = vena cava, R.A. = right atrium, R.V. = right ventricle, L.V. = left ventricle, L.A. = left atrium, P.V. = pulmonary veins.

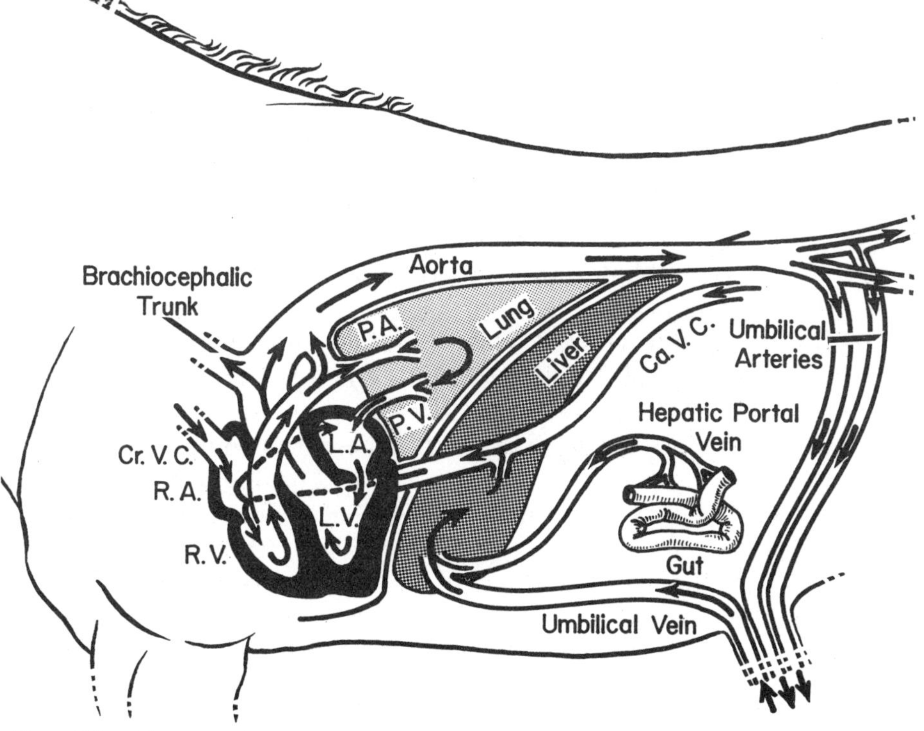

Fig. 28   The circulation of blood before birth. See the text for details. Abbreviations are as in Fig. 27. P.A. = pulmonary artery, Ca. V.C. = vena cava.

much of the blood entering the right atrium simply shunts through an opening (the foramen ovale) into the left atrium, bypassing the lungs. The blood passes from the left atrium to the left ventricle and is, then, pumped out through the aorta to supply the fetal organs and tissues with oxygen and to remove carbon dioxide. The "used" blood then leaves the fetus through the umbilical arteries to reach the placenta. Here it gives up the carbon dioxide and acquires a fresh supply of oxygen. Some blood does pass from the right atrium to the right ventricle and thence through the pulmonary artery to the lung, supplying oxygen and nutrients for the development of the lungs. If too much blood enters the pulmonary artery, however, some of it will be shunted through another by-pass, the ductus arteriosus, from the pulmonary artery to the aorta.

These two bypasses, the foramen ovale and the ductus arteriosus, close at birth, and the pattern of the circulation changes to the postnatal type. Carbon dioxide laden blood returns from the organs and tissues to the right atrium, passes into the right ventricle and, by way of the pulmonary artery, reaches the lungs. The carbon dioxide is released into the air spaces of the lung and oxygen is picked up from those same air spaces.

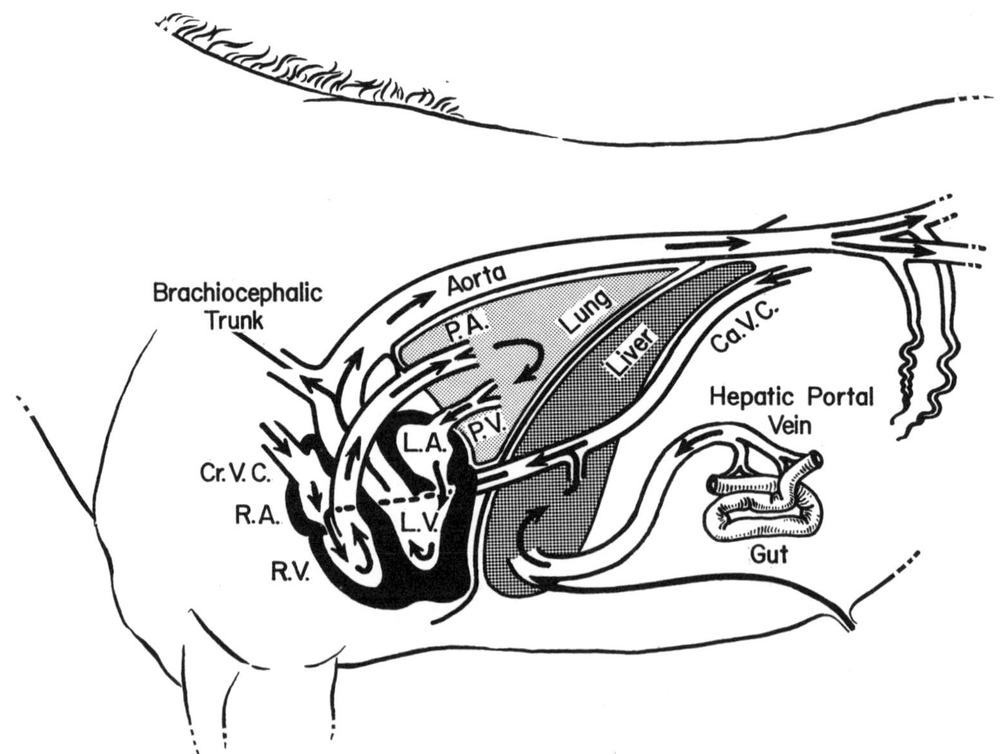

Fig. 29   Circulation of blood after birth.

The blood moves through the pulmonary veins to the left atrium, then the left ventricle and out the aorta.

During fetal life, the blood is, obviously, a mixture of oxygenated and nonoxygenated red cells because blood from the umbilical veins (full of oxygen) mixes in the right atrium with nonoxygenated blood returning to the heart from the tissues and organs of the fetus. From the right atrium this mixed blood travels in the aorta, as described, both to the fetal organs and tissues as well as to the umbilical arteries for return to the placenta. Mixed blood is normal during fetal life but should not be present after birth. The arterial blood should be red, full of oxygen, while the venous blood is blue, poor in oxygen. One of the first signs, then, that a foal may have a heart defect, allowing the mixing of venous and arterial blood, is a bluish color of the mucous membranes rather than the normal pinkish red. A second, clear sign is that the foal has difficulty breathing following even slight exertion. The mixed blood does not have enough oxygen to supply the tissues with the increased demands of exertion. The foal with such a defect, mixed blood, breathes rapidly, attempting to make up the oxygen deficit.

If such signs are observed, a veterinarian should examine the foal. That examination will include listening to the heart with a stethoscope in order to detect abnormal sounds (murmurs). It is often very difficult to determine the precise nature of the heart problem with the stethoscope alone. The examiner will know that a defect is present but only highly sophisticated procedures can reveal the type of defect. No matter what that defect, however, the foal has no chance of becoming a working animal. A word of caution: some foal and young horse hearts do make strange sounds even though there is nothing at all wrong. If in doubt, an expert in heart disease should be consulted.

ARRHYTHMIAS

There is a large group of heart disorders known as arrhythmias. This means that the electrical impulses which regulate the beating of the heart are, for some reason, irregular. Very little is known about the cause of these irregularities, and it is often difficult to decide whether they are clinically significant or not. Again, if there is any trouble, a heart specialist should be summoned. The practising veterinarian cannot be a specialist in everything, but he has colleagues who are, and the heart is a very specialized organ indeed.

BACTERIAL ENDOCARDITIS

A bacterial infection localizing on one of the valves of the heart is called bacterial endocarditis (endo means lining and carditis inflammation of the heart; inflammation of the lining of the heart). The bacterium responsible is, as usual, a streptococcus. It localizes either on the valve between the left atrium and ventricle or the valve between the left ventricle and the aorta. The bacteria enter through a cut, wound or from an abscess somewhere else in the body and travel to the heart in the bloodstream. The clinical signs are a characteristic fluctuating fever, general depression ("looks sick"), and swelling of the tissues of the legs and the undersurface of the body with edema fluid. This fluid accumulates in the tissue because the flow of blood into and out of the heart is slowed because of improper heart action as the result of the endocarditis. The details of edema formation are complex and rather beyond our present scope. The veterinarian can diagnose this condition with considerable accuracy, using the stethoscope and other clinical findings. Fortunately endocarditis is not very common in horses because it is very difficult to treat satisfactorily. Massive doses of penicillin have to be given for a long time, and the prognosis is always guarded.

MYOCARDITIS

Focal or widespread involvement of the heart muscle itself by infection is called myocarditis (myo = muscle). While it is known that streptococci can do this, they are surely not the only cause. Influenza infection and strangles infection can cause localized foci of myocarditis. Viruses are known to cause myocarditis in many species, but there is no information available about such infections in the horse. Myocarditis, as a clinical problem is less common than endocarditis, which is fortunate because it is a quick killer leaving little or no time for treatment.

CORONARY ARTERY DISEASE

Disease of the coronary arteries, so common and important in the human, is virtually nonexistent in the horse. Bloodworm larvae (see Chapter 9) can crawl into the coronary arteries and obstruct them, but that is uncommon and usually the damage is not significant.

ATRIAL FIBRILLATION

This disease of the heart is apparently rather common in horses. The name simply means that the atria, instead of contracting and relaxing in a normal, rhythmical fashion, beat away in a haphazard, irregular manner (fibrillation). The nonworking horse may show no clinical evidence that it is afflicted. When put to work, however, the animal does not do as well as expected. Careful examination with the stethoscope usually allows the diagnosis to be made. It can be difficult, in any given case, however, and expert assistance may be needed. Once diagnosed, the condition can be treated successfully in many horses. The drug used, though, is very toxic and should be administered only under the supervision of someone thoroughly experienced in its use. The cause of the condition is not known but, like roaring and wobbles, seems to go with larger horses.

RUPTURE OF THE AORTA

The horse is somewhat peculiar in his propensity to tear holes in his major blood vessel, the aorta. Older stallions, in particular, may rupture the aorta close to the heart and either die immediately or develop heart failure. When the left ventricle contracts, a column of blood is ejected into the aorta. When the ventricle relaxes, right after the contraction, the column of blood may recoil against the valves between the aorta and ventricle (aortic valves) with such force that the aorta is literally torn away from its attachment to the ventricle. The question, of course, is what makes this recoil so powerful that it disrupts tissue. While a number of factors are involved, one set of circumstances is of particular interest in practical terms.

Most such ruptures are in older stallions and occur during the early part of the breeding season. I have only seen one aortic rupture of this type in the mare. In fact, many cases occur immediately after the stallion covers his first mare of the season. One may reasonably postulate that the extreme excitement of breeding causes a marked elevation of blood pressure. This rise in pressure may be caused by sudden constriction of the peripheral blood vessels. Such constriction causes increased resistance to the movement of blood out of the left ventricle, and, in turn, leads to greater recoil or rebound of the moving column of blood.

In practical terms the stallion is not ready for the cardiovascular "stress" demanded by the breeding process. After being idle in every way for many months, he suddenly is driven to a peak of excitement and stress. With increasing age it is important that the stallion be regularly and properly exercised throughout the year in order to be ready for the breeding season.

This lesson may be emphasized by the following true story: I performed an autopsy on a stallion who had died in this manner. After explaining the findings to the middle-aged farm manager, he looked at me for a long moment and said, "Doc, I'm no spring chicken myself, and I quit playing golf five years ago. I just decided I done made my last cover!"

The aorta may rupture in other areas as well, and I have seen a few cases of rupture of other major blood vessels such as the pulmonary artery. All of these ruptures are quickly fatal and less common than the old stallion ruptures discussed above.

ELECTROCARDIOGRAM

The electrocardiogram is a recording of the electrical pulses moving through the heart muscle. The electrical signal is generated in a special part of the heart called the sinoatrial node and spreads through the heart by way of a special conducting system. The regular, steady pulsing of this electrical impulse regulates the rhythmical contraction and relaxation of the heart muscle. This electrical activity can be picked up by electrodes placed on the skin and recorded on a paper tape for study. The ECG, as it is known, is very helpful in evaluating the condition of the heart muscle and its conducting system. Its interpretation, however, is a matter for experts, and they often don't agree!

7

LIVER AND PANCREAS

The liver is one of the most important and interesting of all the organs in the horse organ collection. It is responsible for a variety of vital functions, including the formation of albumin (a major blood protein), storage of sugars, metabolism of fats, the formation of fibrin which is an important blood-clot protein, and detoxification of toxic materials which may appear in the blood stream. From this incomplete list, it is clear that significant disease or damage to the liver can lead to serious consequences for the entire animal body. The horse can be thankful there are relatively few serious diseases that affect its liver.

THEILER'S DISEASE

Theiler's disease, also known as serum hepatitis, is a total and massive destruction of the liver. The onset of clinical signs is sudden and almost always violent. One of the major liver functions mentioned above, detoxification of noxious substances, is lost. Ammonia is produced in the body as a result of protein metabolism. The liver normally converts this ammonia to urea, a less toxic product which can be excreted by the kidney. If the liver cannot perform this conversion, free ammonia will circulate in increasing quantities in the bloodstream. Ammonia damages the cells of the brain, particularly the cells in the cerebrum. This damage leads to the major clinical sign of mania. The horse usually cannot be caught and runs wildly without direction or sense, crashing through fences, walls or any other obstacle. When so afflicted the animal is extremely dangerous, and no attempt should be made to restrain it.

Death is only hours away, and the liver so totally destroyed that no hope for recovery can be entertained.

The cause of this terrible disease is not known. It is known that it usually, though not invariably, follows 30 to 90 days after the injection of a raw horse protein into a horse. Roughly one out of a thousand horses given a vaccine made in horses or containing horse tissue, or hormone preparations derived from horses, or an antiserum made in horses can be expected to come down with Theiler's disease. The common preparations of this nature still in use are tetanus antitoxin and pregnant mare serum. Whether the liver is destroyed by an allergic reaction or because of a virus present in the horse serum is not known. Experimental study is obviously not feasible, with present knowledge, since only one in a thousand animals are afflicted. Prevention is the obvious answer. Do not give sera or other preparations which have been made in or derived from horses.

You may well have thrown up your hands. How does one get along without tetanus antitoxin since it is known that horses can die of tetanus? The answer is tetanus toxoid injections given on a regular schedule to horses just as they are to humans (those who work with horses should also have those injections!). I hope this point is very clear. If you own a horse, and it has not received tetanus toxoid, stop reading and call your veterinarian. When an injury occurs, a booster toxoid injection can be given to bolster the horse's immunity, and the use of antitoxin completely avoided.

PLANT POISONING

In some areas of this country and other parts of the world plant toxins are an important cause of liver disease in horses. Crotalaria and Senecio are the main offenders. These plants contain a toxin called pyrrolizidine alkaloid. If the horse eats a significant amount of plant material containing this toxin, liver cells will be damaged and destroyed. As the liver tries to repair this damage, scar tissue is laid down instead of normal new cells, and cirrhosis (scarring) of the liver occurs. Gradually and insidiously, more and more liver is replaced by scar tissue until the day, which may be months after exposure to the plant, when there is not enough normal liver remaining, and the horse shows clinical signs of liver failure.

These clinical signs can be identical to those of Theiler's disease—mania. A number of cases, however, will show marked depression rather than mania. In either case, the affected horse almost invariably dies. Free ammonia may be the responsible compound here as in Theiler's disease. The depression may be related to the gradual rise of blood ammonia concentrations (the cells becoming used to it up to a point) as opposed to the mania induced by sudden increases in ammonia as in Theiler's.

There is no treatment, obviously, once symptoms appear. The liver has been destroyed, and the animal cannot live long without a liver. Again, prevention is the answer. If you live in an area where poisonous plants occur (you can find that out from the agricultural college or county agent), you should have an expert coach you on recognizing them. If present, the plants should be removed from pastures and hayfields or the horses moved. The danger is greatest in dry years or on played-out, over-stocked pasturage. Horses usually will not eat poisonous plants unless forced to do so because of poor grazing.

PANCREAS

The pancreas of the horse is rarely the site of significant disease. Most of the damage that occurs is the result of migration of strongyle worm larvae. If enough larvae migrate, acute pancreatitis develops. This acute reaction, however, is apparently not associated with clinical signs of illness. With continued exposure to the larvae, a chronic, scarring type of damage occurs, and this may cause clinical signs. The signs are not specific, and the clinical diagnosis can be very difficult. The animal loses weight and becomes emaciated despite eating voraciously. There may be generalized loss of hair with or without intense itching (a sign strongly suggestive but not diagnostic of pancreatic disease). There is no treatment. The horse is doomed and yet another case is made for proper worming programs!

Diabetes is rare. So-called sugar diabetes (diabetes mellitus) is the result of insufficient production of insulin by the pancreas and may be seen together with the chronic worm disease mentioned above. A more common form of diabetes in the horse is known as diabetes insipidus. There is excessive water intake and urination because of destruction of that part of the pituitary gland which produces the hormone controlling the excretion of water by the kidney (antidiuretic hormone). The cause, in the horse, is almost invariably a tumor of the pituitary gland known as an intermediate lobe adenoma. This tumor occurs in old horses and, apparently, most frequently in mares. The expansion of the tumor destroys part of the pituitary and presses on the brain. Its presence may be deduced from the following clinical signs: either obesity or emaciation (depending on how much of brain is damaged), frequent urination and increased water consumption (stall and bedding constantly wet and water bucket always empty), an excessive amount of hair which is not shed out normally in the spring of the year. The latter is usually the first clinical

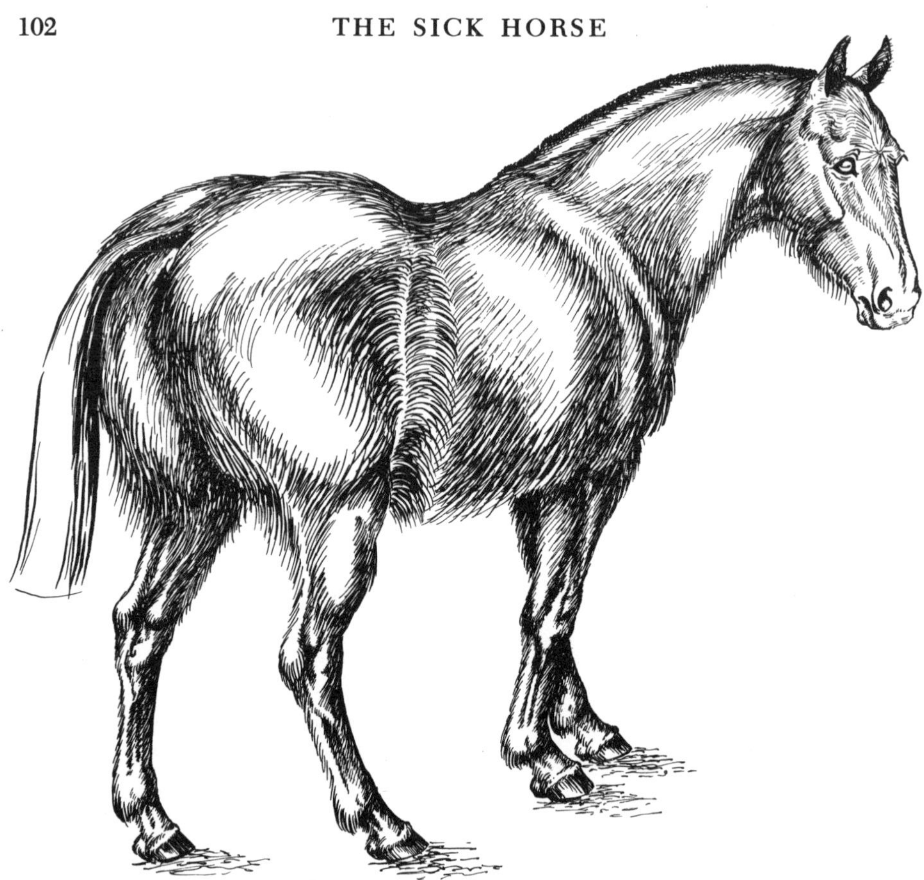

Fig. 30 A very hairy horse as result of a tumor of the pituitary gland.

sign. The animal does not shed out and may, indeed, retain the winter haircoat throughout the summer. While afflicted animals can live for some time, there is no treatment, and death is inevitable.

8
URINARY SYSTEM

This is one of the great organ systems of the horse (Fig. 31). Practically nothing goes wrong with it!

Some twenty years ago I spent several summers working with a veterinarian at a harness track. Almost every day he was asked to treat one or more horses that were "having trouble with their water," as the euphemism went. Being a pure novice with just one year of veterinary school under my belt, I asked him what type of kidney disease horses got that would cause this problem.

His answer: "They don't get kidney disease, but these people think they do, and so I give the horses something that won't do them any harm, and that will keep the trainers from giving them something that might do them some harm."

Now, years later, I hear that horsemen—some horsemen at any rate—still believe in kidney disease. During the interim, I have been a working pathologist trying to determine the cause of illness and death by postmortem examination of some 10,000 or more horses. From this considerable experience of my own and that of my colleagues, it is perfectly clear that disease of the urinary tract—kidneys, ureter, bladder, and urethra—is an extreme rarity in the horse. I have probably seen only 20 examples of significant diseases in the horse's kidneys. That works out to a percentage too small to even calculate.

If this is so, why are some horsemen still convinced that kidney disease and "water" problems are so common? First, horses—particularly stallions and geldings—often put on quite a performance when they urinate, doubling themselves up and groaning for no discernible reason.

Second, the urine of the horse normally contains considerable

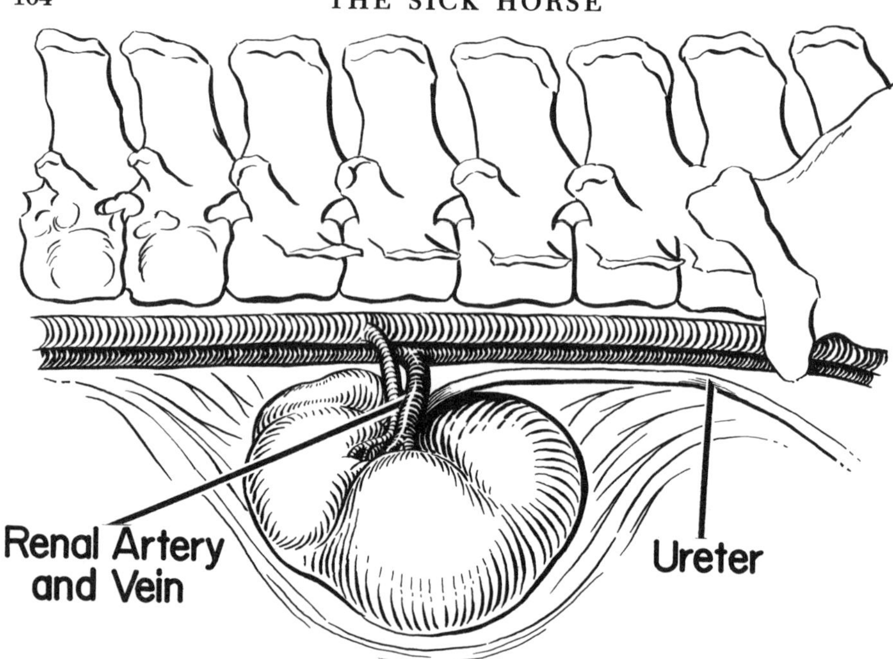

Fig. 31   Kidney located just below backbone. The ureter takes urine from the kidney to the urinary bladder.

quantities of mucus which are produced by cells lining the urinary tract. This is normally clear and not apparent on casual examination. If, however, the horse does not urinate for awhile, such as while being ridden, then when he does urinate, the mucus might have changed to a cloudy, turbid appearance. That isn't abnormal. It simply means·that he has not emptied his bladder for awhile.

A third and singularly important reason for this erroneous belief in kidney disease is sore back. Certainly, in the human, several companies make a great deal of money selling kidney pills to relieve sore back. Most of the time a sore back is probably not at all related to the kidneys. Kidney disease makes people very sick indeed with more than just a sore back!

In the horse, one might think that the back is sore because when you run your fingers along the back, or squeeze the back firmly, the horse bends his belly down toward the ground, moving into a sway-backed position. Actually, this is a normal reflex in the horse, and is called the *spina prominens reflex*. It varies in how obvious it is from horse to horse, but is normally present in all horses.

To really show this, run the point of a ballpoint pen lightly down the back from withers to croup on either side of the top line. You will really see the back bend! Try this on a number of horses and you will see that it is a normal reaction. If the horse *does not* react to the pen pressure, then you can begin to think about sore back!

Now that I have said all this about how few cases of kidney disease there are, I want to note two types that do occur. Horses that are overworked and overheated can develop heat exhaustion to one degree or another. This causes breakdown of red blood cells; and the pigment, hemoglobin, derived from that breakdown, will clog up in the kidneys and might cause kidney disease anywhere from five to ten days later.

The second condition is old-fashioned "Monday morning sickness" or azoturia. For reasons still not completely understood, horses rested for a few days but kept on a full grain ration might develop severe muscle damage, particularly of the large croup muscles. The damaged muscles release a pigment, myoglobin, which is very similar to hemoglobin. This pigment, again, can clog up the kidneys and cause fatal kidney disease.

Finally, many horses in the initial stages of colicky pain arising in the abdomen might strain and tighten the abdomen trying to relieve the pain. While doing so, some dribbles of urine might be squeezed out, and the immediate reaction is that the horse is having trouble passing water. You'd better believe it is colic and get help fast. Horses with kidney disease do not strain in this fashion.

Let us hope, then, that this old ghost is laid to rest once more. But he will probably rise again, I'm sure, and for the wrong reasons.

There is one unique and horrible disease of the urinary system which has been seen in the southwestern section of the United States. A toxin produced by the Spanish fly beetle is eaten by the horse, and this toxin literally tears the urinary system to pieces with necrosis and bleeding. The toxin, *cantharidin*, damages many tissues but is excreted through the urinary system and does the most damage there.

The Spanish fly beetle infests irrigated alfalfa with great glee. When the alfalfa is cut, dried and made into hay in the old way, the beetles leave the drying legume, and no harm comes to the horse eating the hay. When hay crushers came into widespread use (they crush the stalks of the fresh-cut alfalfa and hasten drying), they crushed the beetles along with the alfalfa stalks. Horses eating the hay, then, ingested the crushed beetles and their toxin, and the damage was done.

Cystitis, inflammation of the urinary bladder, is not common in horses. When affected, the horse will show pain, dribbling of urine with scalding of the rearquarters of mares and the sheath of geldings or stallions. Laboratory examination of the urine will confirm that cystitis is present. So far as I know there are only two causes of cystitis in the horse: stones (calculi) in the bladder and damage to the nerves which go to the bladder. The first cause is rare and seen almost exclusively in very old horses. The second is slightly more common. Damage to the nerves may be associated with neuritis of the cauda equina, myelitis of the spinal cord and other neurological conditions.

When the nerves to the bladder are damaged, the muscle of the bladder is partially or completely paralyzed. With such paralysis, urine remains in the lumen of the bladder for protracted periods and undergoes decomposition. The products of this decomposition irritate the bladder and cause inflammation.

In the case of stones, surgical treatment may be helpful, but there is little or nothing one can do about damaged nerves.

9
WORMS

This is the most important single chapter in this book. Worms and gnats and other little beasties that go bump in the night may not be glamorous and exciting, but they are the most insidious and destructive of all the enemies of the horse.

INSECTS

The common housefly is more nuisance than threat to the horse with the exception of its role as vector for the roundworm, *Habronema*. There are three species of Habronema: *H. musca*, *H. majus*, and *Draschia megastoma*. The eggs of the worms are ingested by houseflies feeding on horse manure. The eggs hatch into larvae inside the fly, and either the fly or the larvae can be swallowed by the horse. The larvae travel down the esophagus to the stomach and develop in the lining of the stomach wall causing the lining to become chronically inflamed and form nodules. If a sufficient number of larvae invade the stomach, significant damage may be done and clinical illness appear. The signs of illness are nonspecific: loss of weight and general "poor doing". One specific and dramatic sign sometimes associated with widespread, chronic inflammation of the stomach is hypocalcemic tetany. Apparently insufficient hydrochloric acid is produced by the damaged stomach lining, and calcium taken in the food cannot be properly ionized (broken down into small "bits" which can be absorbed through the gut wall). With insufficient absorption of calcium, the blood level of calcium drops, and the horse will have attacks of muscle spasm and collapse. Calcium is necessary for proper muscle activity. The veterinarian can "cure" the attack by administering calcium intravenously, but it will often recur. While there is insufficient evidence to say that such tetanic attacks are always caused by Habronema infestation, the possibility should be kept in mind and affected horses wormed to rid them of Habronema.

Not satisfied with damaging the stomach, the housefly and its fellow-traveling habronema larvae can produce significant damage to the skin of the horse. Any slight cut or wound will, as everyone knows, attract the feeding attentions of the housefly. While it feeds on the wound, the Habronema larvae can escape from the fly into the wound. The larvae invade the tissues in and around the wound, and the body reacts with a chronic inflammation, forming a lump or nodule (just as in the stomach). Often the original wound will have healed by the time the nodule appears, and it may seem as if a tumor is developing. These nodules may be quite a nuisance and can be dealt with by surgical means or by the use of a paste containing drugs which kill the offending larvae.

The best strategy, of course, is prevention. The flies should be either killed or screened away from the horses. Any small cut or abrasion should be dealt with promptly, particularly in the southern states where flies and, therefore, larvae are numerous.

The *stable fly* is a biting fly and can cause considerable irritation and restlessness in a band of horses. It, too, can carry the Habronema larvae. *Horse flies, deer flies* and others of their ilk are bloodsuckers and can be most annoying to horse and man. The horsefly, in particular, is said to be the transmitter of equine infectious anemia virus (more about that one later).

Blackflies, mosquitos, sand flies and *gnats* are not of great importance with stabled horses. It is possible, however, for these minute blood-suckers to cause great harm and even to kill horses that are kept in the open. Millions of gnats attacking a horse all through the night can deplete the animal of a considerable volume of blood and may directly or indirectly be the cause of death. Mosquitos are of significance as vectors for the transmission of certain virus diseases of the nervous system.

Flies, midges and other insects may be one cause of an allergic inflammation of the skin during the summer months. This condition, *summer eczema,* can be very unsightly and annoying to the horse. While difficult to diagnose precisely, it should be a rule of thumb to protect all horses with skin lesions from insects and flies. That may cure the problem or, at least, protect the skin from secondary damage (as by habronema).

Screworms, the larvae of certain flies, can be a severe problem in the southern states, invading superficial skin wounds and causing a severe, chronic inflammation and ulceration of the skin.

The face fly, *Musca autumnalis,* collects on the horse's face, usually around the nose and eyes. While they may not do direct damage, they are a great annoyance to the horse.

Lice can and do infest horses and can do considerable damage. As they bite into the skin to feed, they irritate, causing the horse to rub and further damage the area, allowing secondary infection to occur. If heavily infested the horse may lose considerable blood and become debilitated. No one likes to think of lice on their horses, but it does happen and stabled animals, in particular, should be checked regularly for the wee brutes.

Ticks are rarely a problem. The spinose ear tick may infest the ears in the southwest United States and other dry areas. They cause irritation and itching.

There are three mites that can infest horses: *Sarcoptes, Psoroptes*, and *Chorioptes*. They all cause a nasty dermatitis (inflammation of the skin). Sarcoptes usually starts on the neck, shoulder and head. Psoroptes prefers the base of the tail, the mane and just beneath the foretop. Chorioptes sets up housekeeping on the rear feet and legs. If there should be a skin problem located in these areas, veterinary help should be summoned immediately. The mites are very contagious and difficult to treat, causing considerable damage to a number of horses before they can be controlled.

While simple observation would seem to be all that is necessary to know that flies and gnats and such winged critters are about, it is surprising how often they are overlooked and/or discounted. Little fellows like gnats and midges attack during the early evening hours when the human is in the house and the horse out on the marsh. The horse may be frazzled and worn the next morning from the night's working over by the legions of winged hypodermic needles.

For all of these insects, rigid stable hygiene is one obvious answer. Insects can be controlled with poisons, but these should be supplemented with screening and removal of manure a considerable distance from barns. Light traps and old-fashioned sticky paper are effective. Horses living in endemic insect areas should be stabled at night in screened barns. Nothing will be said here about the drugs which can be used to prevent and treat. New drugs and compounds of old ones come out daily, and anything I might say would be out of date by the time you read it.

INTERNAL PARASITES

Here come the badies! The horse has a multitude of wormy creatures that choose to live with and inside him. Some are quite harmless, while others are lethal. As I have said before, and shall again, there is nothing more important, more destructive and more costly than some of those creatures we now have to discuss.

STOMACH

The other important roundworm of the stomach, apart from Habronema, is *Trichostrongylus axei*. This worm primarily infests cattle, sheep and goats and is usually only found in horses living in association with these species. While light infestations are of no importance, heavy infestations can cause an acute inflammation of the stomach (acute gastritis). If you've had acute indigestion, you'll know how the horse feels. Clinical signs are nonspecific: discomfort, loss of weight, etc. Fortunately, these worms are readily removed by the same drugs used to control strongyles (see below).

The commonest parasites of the stomach are the larval stages of the bot flies. There are three types: *Gasterophilus nasalis*, *G. intestinalis* and *G. hemorrhoidalis*. The first two are most common in the United States. Bot flies, during the summer, lay their eggs on hairs either around the mouth or on the legs of the horse. The larvae hatch and crawl into the horse's mouth, down the esophagus and into the stomach. They attach in the stomach and undergo several moults (stages in their development) before becoming full-sized, third stage larvae. The latter may remain in the stomach over the winter and pass out in the feces the following spring to develop into adult flies which begin the cycle over again. That may seem a strange sort of life to lead but wait until we come to some of the others!

Horsemen worry a great deal more about bots than is necessary. The adult flies bite and worry horses as they go about their egg-laying activities. (How would you like a fly laying eggs on your head!) The larvae in the stomach certainly do no good, but the amount of damage they produce is actually quite minor, and most horses are able to tolerate their presence very well.

Control, first of all, is to reduce fly propulations. The egg cases (small oval yellow things stuck to the hairs of the legs) can be clipped off or simply washed regularly with warm water. The warm water causes the eggs to hatch prematurely, and the larvae die before they can reach the protection of the stomach. Traditionally, horses are "botted," in temperate climates, after the first killing frost, and the treatment is repeated in a few weeks to kill any remaining larvae or late arrivals. Botting is the administration, by stomach tube, of a drug which will kill the bot larvae. There are a variety of drugs available, but those containing carbon disulfide still seem to be best.

Small Intestine

There are several parasites of the small intestine which are of little importance. Two species of *coccidia* may live in the upper part of the small intestine, but the infestation seems to be self-curing and causes no illness or clinical signs. A tiny worm, *Strongyloides*, may infest the small intestine, and, again, is self-curing and causes no clinical signs. Some people believe that this worm causes diarrhea in the young foal because the worms may be found in the feces. That is insufficient evidence, however, and all evidence indicates that the worm is inocuous.

There are three tapeworms that can infest the small and large intestine. *Anoplocephala perfoliata* lives in the cecum and, on occasion, in the lower end of the small intestine. A. *magna* and A. *mammillana* are much

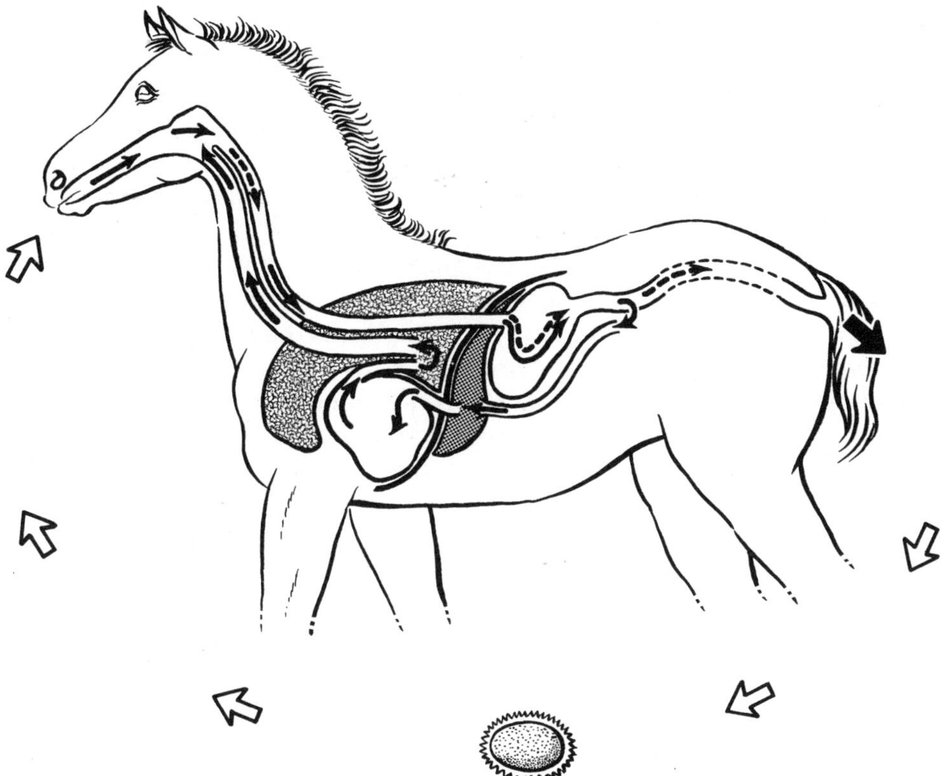

Fig. 32   Life cycle of the ascarid. The eggs are picked up with grass, swallowed, and pass down the esophagus to the stomach and small intestine. They migrate from the intestine through the liver and lung, are coughed up into the throat and reswallowed. Once again in the small intestine they develop into egg-laying adults.

less common and live entirely in the small intestine. These flatworms cause small erosions by attaching to the gut lining. They are rarely, if ever, present in sufficient numbers to cause clinical disease. The usual worm treatments do not remove tapeworms. If a heavy infestation is suspected, specific drugs must be used.

Parascaris equorum, the large, white roundworm of the horse, is a very dangerous parasite for the young foal. Any pasture which has ever known a horse will be contaminated with ascarid eggs, and these eggs are very long-lived and hardy. The foal, a curious creature, begins to nibble about during the first day or so after birth. Ascarid eggs are picked up and swallowed. The eggs hatch in the foal, and the larvae migrate widely through the organs before returning to the small intestine to become egg-laying adults. The life cycle of the ascarid is shown in Figure 32.

The larvae migrate through the liver and lungs, causing areas of necrosis and inflammation which inhibit the normal growth of the foal as well as providing weak points for secondary bacterial infection. The adult worms in the small intestine, however, are the most dangerous. They can induce a variably severe and persisting diarrhea and, when present in large numbers, can obstruct and cause perforation of the intestine. The latter, of course, leads to a fatal peritonitis.

Interestingly, as the foal matures into an adult, resistance to ascarid infestation develops, and it is rare to see significant ascarid infestation in adult horses. Occasionally, however, an older mare or one with a chronic disease (such as pleuritis) may lose that resistance and acquire a substantial ascarid infestation. Such older, infested animals can serve as a significant source of egg contamination of the pasture. The most important aspect of a worming program for foals is complete and thorough worming of the mares with which those foals associate. We seek to reduce the numbers and availability of eggs on the pasture as much as possible. Worming the foal is necessary but will be that much more effective if the mother is not shedding ascarid eggs in his path.

Large Intestine

There are four members of the family of Strongyle worms that need to be considered: *small strongyles, Strongylus vulgaris, S. edentatus*, and *S. equinus.*

The small strongyles are a group of several different species of worms. They shall be considered as a group, however, since the differences between species, insofar as they effect the horse, are insignificant. What is that effect? In general, small strongyles alone do not cause any specific or well-defined disease or clinical signs. At most, a heavy infestation with these worms may result in slight inappetance and barely detectable change in the feces (slight diarrhea). If carefully weighed and examined, it may be apparent that foals and young horses with heavy infestations are not growing as thriftily and rapidly as expected.

The adults reside on the surface of the large intestinal lining (the mucosa). They do not penetrate the lining, damaging tissue and ingesting blood, as do the large strongyles. They are living, then, almost entirely on food materials within the gut lumen and, in order to damage the horse, would have to be present in enormous numbers.

The major significance of the small strongyles is as an indicator of the presence of the large strongyles: vulgaris, edentatus and equinus. Small numbers of these large strongyles can cause immoderate damage. Because they can be present in small numbers, producing few eggs, they are not readily detected by the routine fecal egg count (see below). Fortunately, whenever large strongyles are present, small strongyles are almost invariably present as well. Therefore, when the fecal egg count rises, the eggs being counted are mainly small strongyle eggs. It is assumed, then, that whenever the total count rises, the large strongyles are increasing along with the small, and that a dangerous situation is developing. Egg production by small strongyles, therefore, serves as a warning sign of dangerous increases in large strongyles. I hate to say anything nice about a worm, but these little guys are doing us a favor!

The principle technique for detecting parasitic infestation of the gut is the fecal egg count. A measured amount of fecal material is diluted with a sugar solution (or something similarly dense) and allowed to stand for a period. The parasite eggs (most of them, though not the tapeworms) float to the top of the dense sugar solution. A sample is taken from the top of the mixture, placed on a microscopic slide and the eggs counted. The total eggs per amount of feces can then be interpreted in terms of the degree of parasite infestation. This technique is neither perfect nor infallible. The counts must be interpreted in terms of the farm, the horses and many environmental and management practises. It is not an exercise for the inexperienced.

Strongylus edentatus and *Strongylus equinus* are two of the three large strongyles. While S. *equinus* infestations are not common, they can be quite devastating for the horse. The effects of the worm on the pancreas have already been described. The larvae ingested with grass pass to the cecum and bore through the wall of the cecum to enter veins by which they travel to the liver. They wander for months in the liver, destroying tissue wherever they go. They finally migrate back through the pancreas to reach the large intestine where they develop into egg-laying adults. Obviously there are a variety of opportunities to do damage during the course of such a migration.

Strongylus edentatus is, on the other hand, not rare. The infective

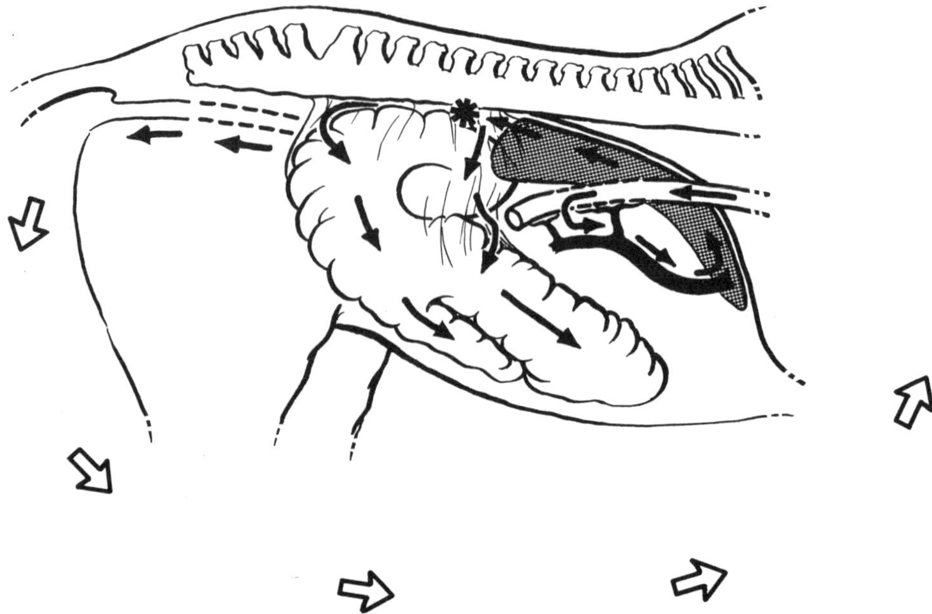

Fig. 33   Life cycle of *S. edentatus*. The infective larvae are swallowed, penetrate the wall of the gut and travel in the portal vein (the dark tube beneath the hatched liver). They migrate in the liver and, then, into the flank (the asterisk). Finally, they return to the large intestine to become adults. *S. equinus* migrates in the same way but returns to the large intestine by way of the pancreas.

larvae live on the grass. The horse eats the grass, and the larvae are swallowed and pass down the gut to the cecum. They bore into the wall of the cecum and, thence, into the veins in the cecal wall. From there they travel in the portal vein to the liver where they wander for months, precisely like *S. equinus*. After their gambol through the liver, they leave and move into the deep layers of the flanks, just beneath the peritoneal lining of the abdomen. Finally, the larvae, which have been moulting and changing, leave the flank, cross the abdominal cavity and bore into the large intestine to become egg-laying adults. In addition to the obvious damage which such migrations can cause, blockage of the cecal veins can lead to a chronically poorly functioning cecum, so-called chronic typhlitis (chronic inflammation of the cecum).

With both edentatus and equinus infestations there may be no overt and outward signs of the damage being done. It is certain, however, that the damage done to the liver, pancreas, or cecum can impair the health and performance capabilities of working horses. The worms may make the difference between the horse that wins and the one that just misses.

We come now to the most devilish, rascally worm of them all: Strongylus vulgaris (the blood worm or red worm). There is so much to say about this wretch that it is difficult to know where to begin!

The eggs of *Strongylus vulgaris* are produced by mature female worms in the large intestine. The eggs pass out with the feces and hatch, on the ground, into infective larvae. The microscopic larvae crawl up on blades of grass and wait to be swallowed by a grazing horse. They quickly pass from the mouth to the lower part of the small intestine and cecum. The larvae burrow through the lining of the gut and enter the small arteries in the wall of the gut. Within these vessels they migrate upward toward the major artery (cranial mesenteric artery) which supplies most of the blood to the intestinal tract. Once they reach this main artery the greatest damage will be done to the horse, and fatal consequences are all too common.

Before reaching the main artery, however, much damage is done. During their burrowing in the wall of the intestine the larvae block small arteries, decreasing the flow of blood to part of the gut wall. If a sufficient number of such small arteries are blocked, the gut will become infarcted

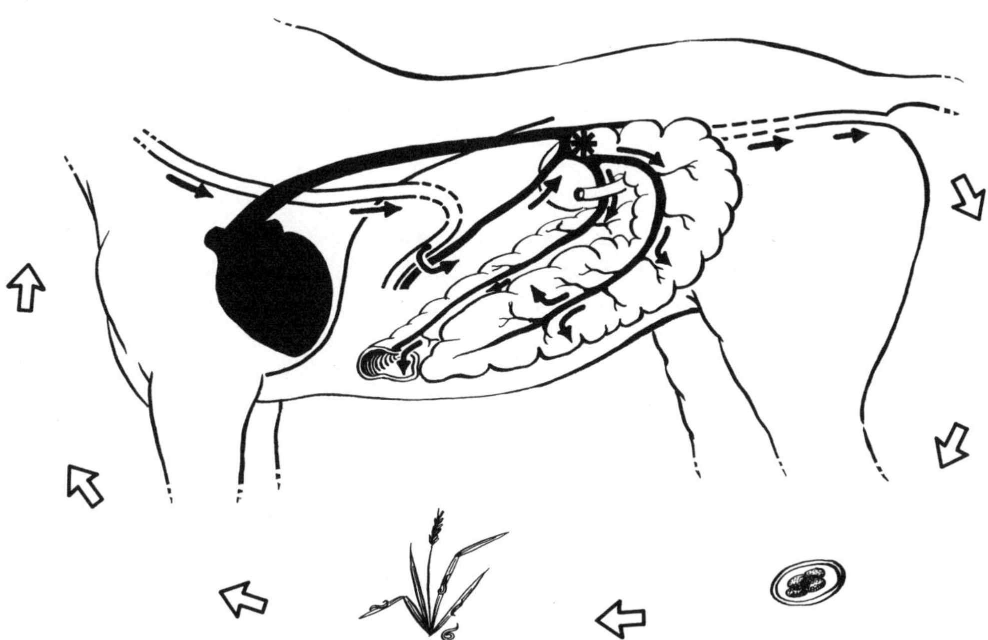

Fig. 34   Life cycle of *S. vulgaris*. The ingested larvae enter the arteries supplying the gut and migrate up the vessels to the cranial mesenteric artery (asterisk). After a period in that vessel they migrate down arteries to enter the large intestine and become adults.

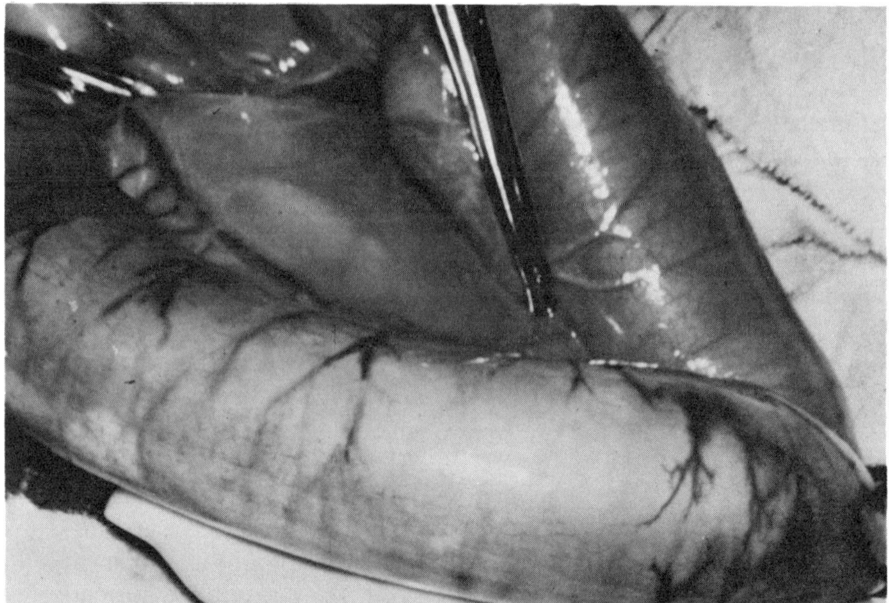

Fig. 35 Infarction, blockage of blood vessels to the small intestine by vulgaris larvae. The dead segment of gut is below center, below the tip of the forceps and lighter in color.

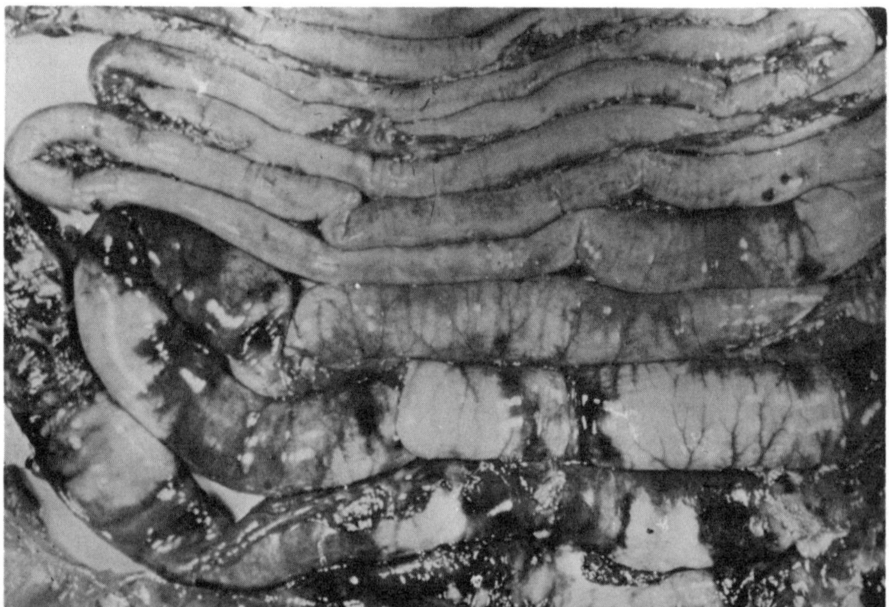

Fig. 36 The whole small intestine of a pony killed by vulgaris. The gut above is normal while the mottled pattern below is the result of infarction.

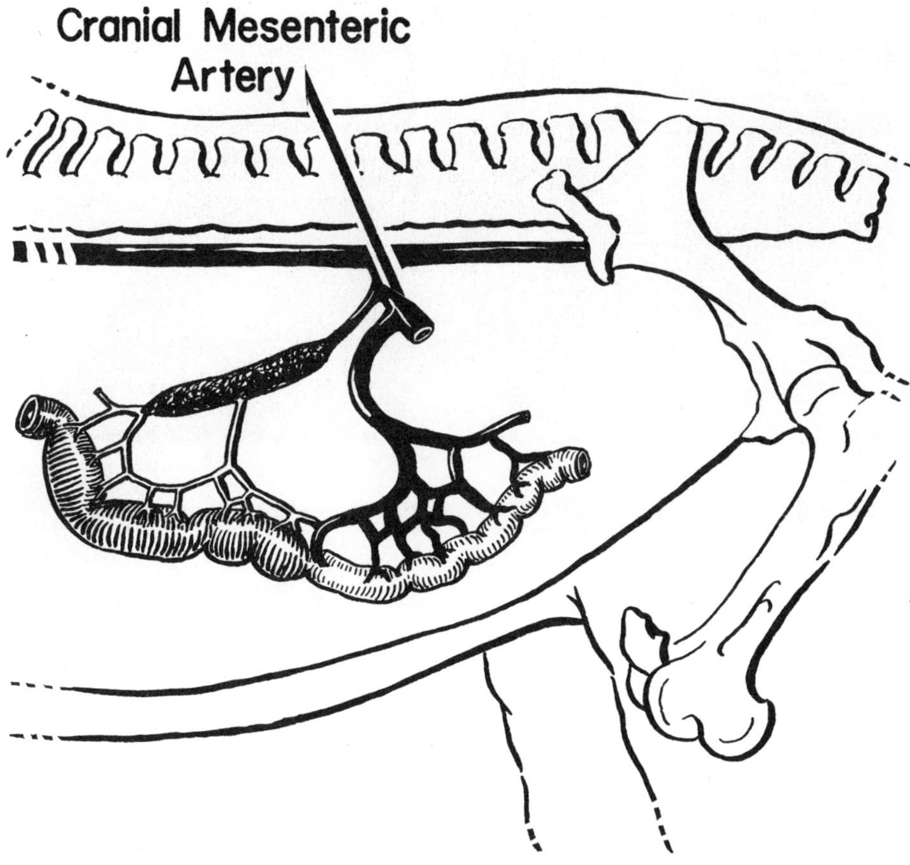

Fig. 37 Schematic drawing showing a thrombus in vessels to the small intestine (to the left) causing infarction of the intestine.

(deprived totally of blood) and die. When the gut dies, food material leaks through the wall into the abdominal cavity and fatal peritonitis is the result.

If some, but not all, vessels are blocked, blood flow will be decreased with a resulting slowing of the normal muscular movement of the gut. This can lead to any one of several types of fatal "twisting" of the gut.

The tissues of the intestinal wall react vigorously to the presence of the larvae and scars will be formed. These scars, with the lovely name of hemamelasma ilei (bloody-black spots on the ileum or gut), can be associated with fatal twisting of the gut and intussusception (telescoping) of the small intestine into the cecum, a nasty and usually (without surgery) fatal event.

These several effects of the bloodworm larvae appear to be dose and

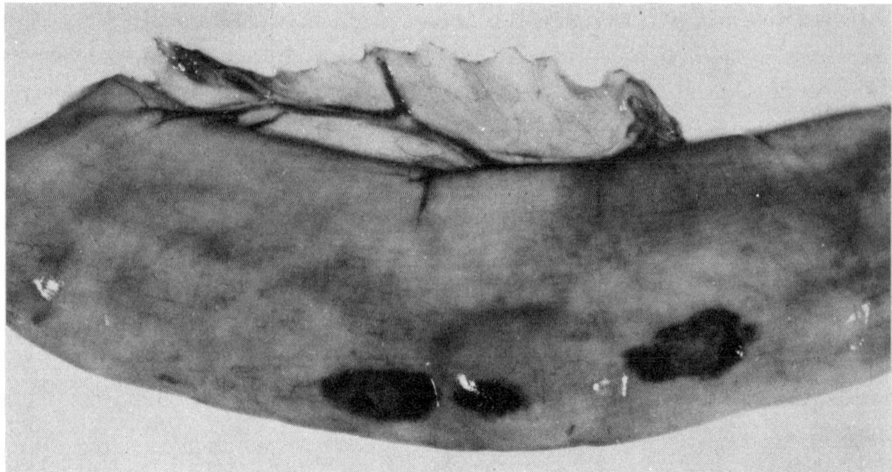

Fig. 38 Scars in the wall of the intestine caused by vulgaris larvae.

time dependent. That is, if only a few larvae are ingested at any one time, relatively little damage may be done. If many larvae enter in a short period of time, there may well be either temporary or complete blockage of blood vessels to the small intestine with twisting or infarction of the gut. If many worms are ingested over a longer period, the cranial mesenteric artery will be severely damaged, and infarction of the large intestine occurs.

The larvae require about three weeks to get from the gut to the cranial mesenteric artery. Once there, the larvae remain for a period. The first time strongyle larvae reach this vessel in the foal, the reaction of the body is nonspecific, simply inflammation as would be elicited by any foreign material. Second and subsequent waves of larvae, however, elicit an allergic inflammatory reaction. The horse has made antibody against the larvae, but, unfortunately, that antibody does not protect the horse. In fact, the antibody, working against the larvae, increases the severity of the damage to the blood vessels.

If, on the first or subsequent invasions, there are a sufficient number of larvae, the artery will be plugged by fibrin (forming a thrombus) and the large intestine completely deprived of blood. The large intestine is, then, infarcted and dies, and the horse dies right along with it. The earliest deaths from this cause are at 28 to 30 days of age. That means that the foal picked up the larvae while nibbling at the grass the day he was born! (It is clear that the larvae do not go from the mare to the fetus within the uterus.)

If the thrombus forming in the cranial mesenteric artery does not plug the vessel completely, it may break off pieces (emboli) which wash down the branches of the artery to shut off segments of the branches causing infarction of portions of the large intestine. Leakage of ingesta through the dead gut wall occurs, and peritonitis finishes the horse.

Assuming that fatal blockages of this sort do not occur, the larvae eventually migrate down the branches of the cranial mesenteric artery, break out into the lumen of the large intestine and become egg-laying adults which start the whole vicious cycle all over again. While in the lumen of the large intestine, the adult worms fasten themselves to the lining of the intestine and take blood from the horse to supply their own needs (thus the name "bloodworm"). Heavy infestations, then, can cause anemia.

That is the usual pattern. Frequently, on their migrations the larvae lose their way and wander at random through the body. They can,

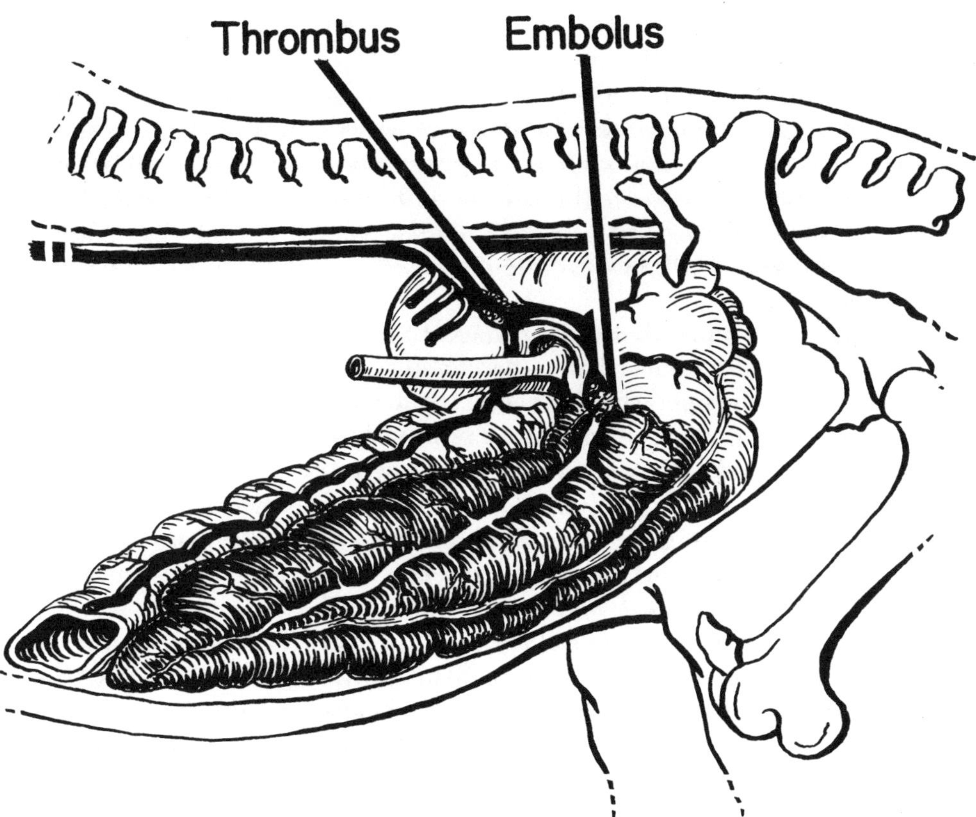

Fig. 39   Infarction of the large intestine (the cecum in this instance) by an embolus which has broken off from a thrombus in the cranial mesenteric artery.

literally, go anywhere: heart, brain, spinal cord, lung, liver, testes. You name it and they can go there. damaging and destroying as they go!

One must admit that these are versatile and protean agents of destruction, an enemy that requires our best vigilance and control. Our tools at present are: 1) fecal egg counts on a regular basis. 2) Pasture management consists of: a) avoiding overstocking, b) regular rotation with cattle or sheep. The latter can "vacuum" many of the infective larvae from the pasture, and the strongyles do not harm these animals. c) Remove manure from the pasture regularly or harrow regularly to break up the manure so that it can dry, killing the larvae. d) Compost all stable manure for four to five years before spreading it on horse pastures. e) Do not graze horses in heavily contaminated areas such as riding stables, show areas, racetracks, etc.

The drugs used in treatment of the bloodworm are called anthelmintics (anti—helminths and strongyles are helminths). I shall not enter into an extended discussion of drugs since, as mentioned before, the situation may be quite different by the time you read this. Horses should be wormed on a regular basis determined by fecal egg counts, rate of stocking, horse traffic (every new horse should be thoroughly wormed before being turned out) and, most importantly, the collaborative judgement of the horseman and the veterinarian. Each farm is different, and the worm control program must reflect those differences. In heavily contaminated, over-stocked areas horses will be wormed every month or, at most, every other month. Less frequent worming may be appropriate for a given situation, but egg counts should be done any month that worming is not done.

It is true that strongyles quickly develop resistance to any given drug if that drug is given over and over again. They should all be used, alternating each time. There can't be too many things to use against the bloodworm. Whatever drug is used, however, should be highly effective against that worm. Many patent wormers knock out small strongyles and, thereby, lower the egg count but are relatively ineffective against *S. vulgaris*. Labels and advertising should be read carefully (it is frequently misleading) and a veterinarian consulted.

Farther down the large intestine there is a relatively innocent worm, *Oxyuris equi*. It lives in or near the anus and cause intense itching of the tail and perineal area. The horse will rub his tail on anything available, leaving much of his tail hair festooned someplace other than his tail. Happily, these worms are readily removed by all the drugs used against strongyles and present no real health or control problem.

Other Worms

Lungworms, *Dictyocaulus*, are not, as a rule, a significant problem in horses. Most infestations are associated with burros. In fact, it is rare to find a burro, at postmortem examination, that does not have some degree of lungworm infestation. The few cases of lungworm infestation that I have seen were in horses kept with burros. Prevention, then, is clear enough! There is a method of treatment for lungworm in cattle, but it has not been tested in horses so far as I know.

A unique roundworm that can cause problems in horses is *Onchocerca cervicalis*. The adult worms live in the ligamentum nuchae, a large, elastic ligament that helps to support the head and neck. Why they choose such a bizarre and out-of-the-way homestead is a mystery. The adults damage the ligament, but this is rarely a clinically significant problem. The adults produce large numbers of offspring called micorfilaria (little hair-like worms) which circulate in the bloodstream and eventually localize in the skin. Apparently, these microfilaria do little harm until they die. The dead larvae incite an inflammatory reaction which appears, clinically, as a loss of hair and swollen, inflammed areas of skin (dermatitis). Lesions caused by the microfilaria usually appear on the lower midline of the belly and on the face, around the eyes. They may localize in the eye itself and, dying there, elicit an inflammation in the eye which is called moon blindness.

There is no absolute way to prevent this type of infestation which manifests itself primarily during the warmer months. Since the microfilaria are apparently transferred from horse to horse by mosquitos, control of those creatures is the obvious strategy. Treatment with certain drugs will kill the microfilaria, but steroids may be necessary to suppress the deleterious effects of the allergic inflammatory reaction induced by the dead microfilaria.

10

GASTROINTESTINAL TRACT

The gastrointestinal tract is a large, complex organ system. Many of the problems associated with this system have already been considered, but a few remain.

Food material taken into the mouth passes down the esophagus to the stomach. The horse's stomach is quite small and holds food material (ingesta) for short periods. Digestion of soluble sugars, proteins, and the absorption of calcium begin here. Roughages, such as grass and hay, leave the stomach and quickly move down the roughly seventy feet of small intestine (duodenum, jejunum, ileum) to the large intestine (the cecum, the first part of the large intestine). During the trip through the small intestine the more soluble proteins and sugars are absorbed through the gut wall into the bloodstream. Most roughage, however, is cellulose, a tough, complex sugar which cannot be digested by the enzymes produced by the intestine and pancreas. In the cecum and ventral colon, however, there is a large, active population of bacteria, protozoa, and fungi which can digest cellulose both for their own use and the use of the host animal. As these organisms break down cellulose, short chain fatty acids (acetic acid, for one) are produced, and these are absorbed and used as energy by the horse. The system is comparable to that of the ruminants (cow, sheep) except that in ruminants the stomach is the site for the microbial breakdown of cellulose.

A great deal of water is used and added to the contents of the cecum and colon during the course of cellulose digestion. Much of that water is

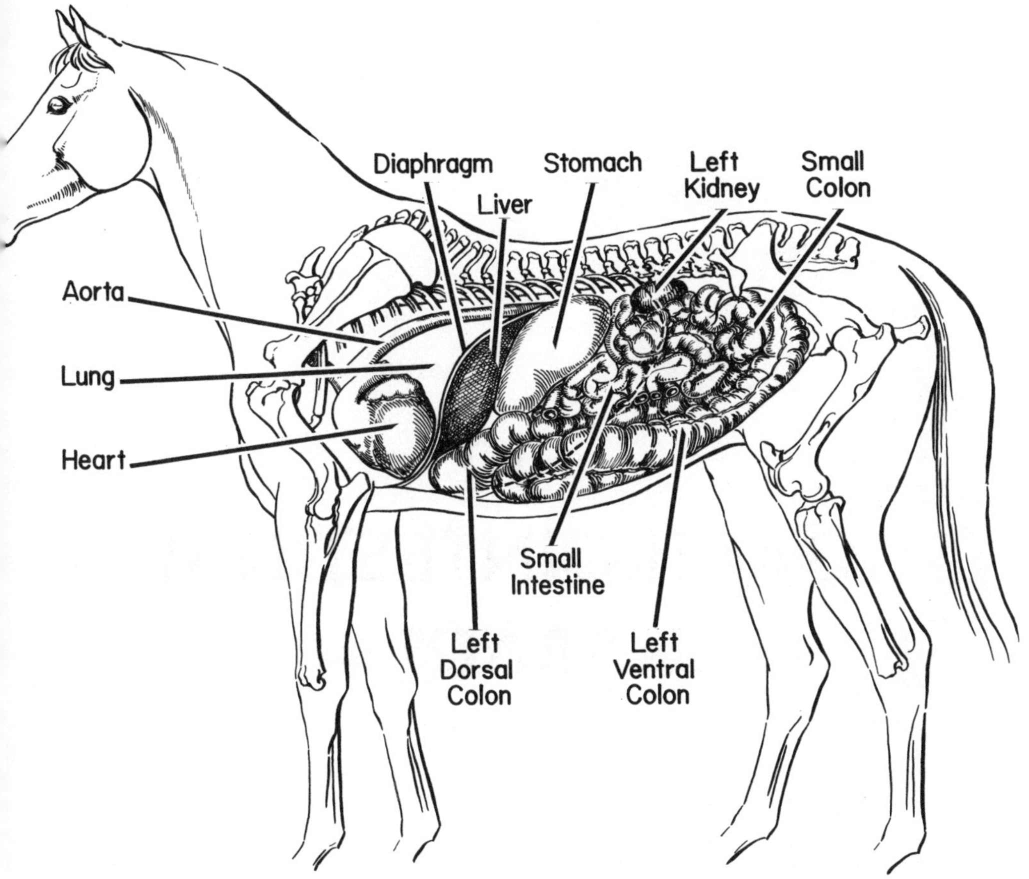

Fig. 40 and 41 **Side views of the arrangement of the viscera (the internal organs) of the horse.**

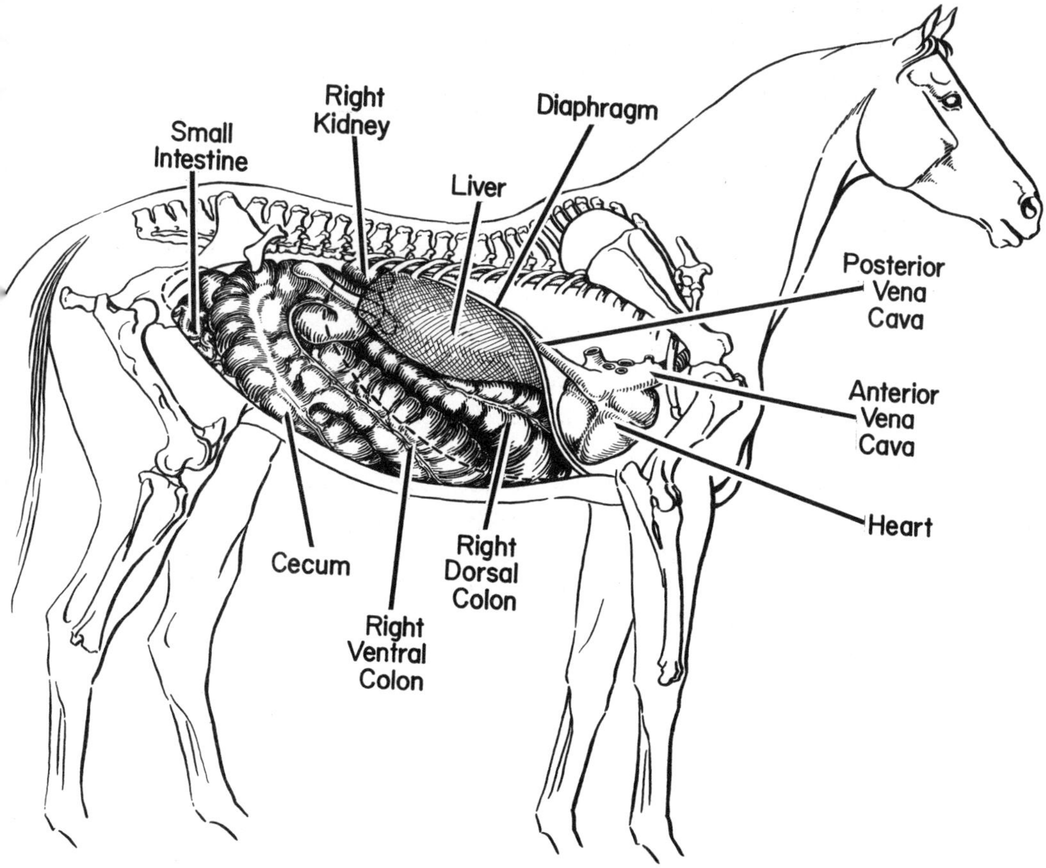

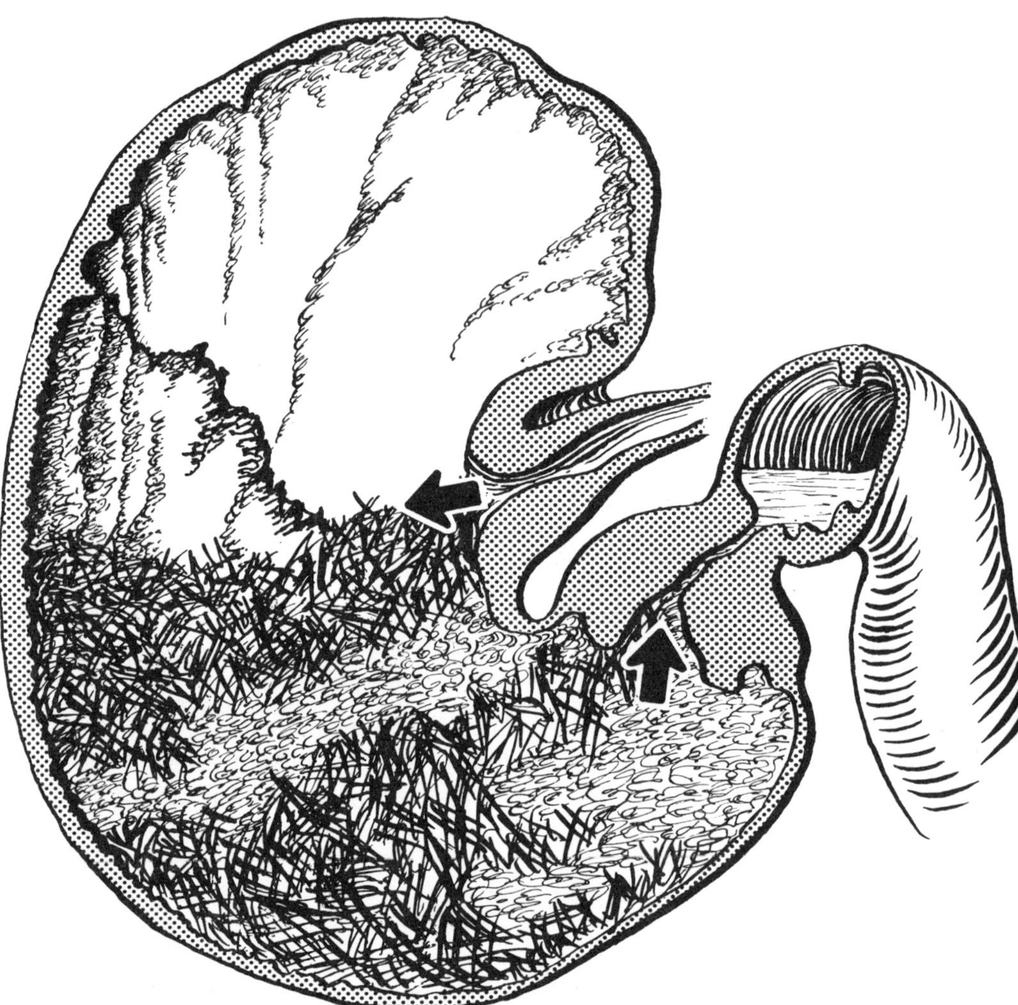

Fig. 42 Side view of the opened stomach of a horse. The upper arrow is the opening of the esophagus into the stomach and the lower arrow the exit into the duodenum. Note that the ingesta lies in layers in the stomach.

resorbed by the lower parts of the colon before the ingesta residues (now called feces) are expelled from the body. Certain of the organisms in the large intestine also produce B vitamins as part of their metabolic processes, and the horse can absorb these vitamins for its own use. This relationship between the horse and the organisms living in its digestive tract is known as a symbiotic relationship. The horse provides a home, warmth, and water for the organisms, and they, in turn, provide fatty acids and vitamins, at least. Even if one cannot ascribe purpose to this relationship, it is a lot nicer than the warfare which goes on between strongyles and the horse.

Food materials such as grain which have little or no cellulose seem to move down the small intestine more slowly than roughage as the soluble sugars, proteins and fats are digested and absorbed.

ESOPHAGUS

The teeth and head will be considered later. The only significant disorder of the esophagus in the horse is *choke*. Food materials or, uncommonly, foreign materials of other sorts accumulate in the esophagus and do not move normally down to the stomach. There are several factors involved. Older horses seem more prone to the problem because of poor, worn teeth and old-age weakness. Poor teeth mean inadequate chewing, and the long, rough hay or forage is more likely to impact in the esophagus.

Dry feed together with an inadequate water supply may predispose to choke. The horse needs water to wash down food and should be allowed to use it. Pelleted feeds can cause choke unless the horse is gradually accustomed to them, and adequate water is always available.

Horses may develop appetites for strange things. Rubber fences and rubber tires used as feed tubs may turn the horse on, and a rubber choke

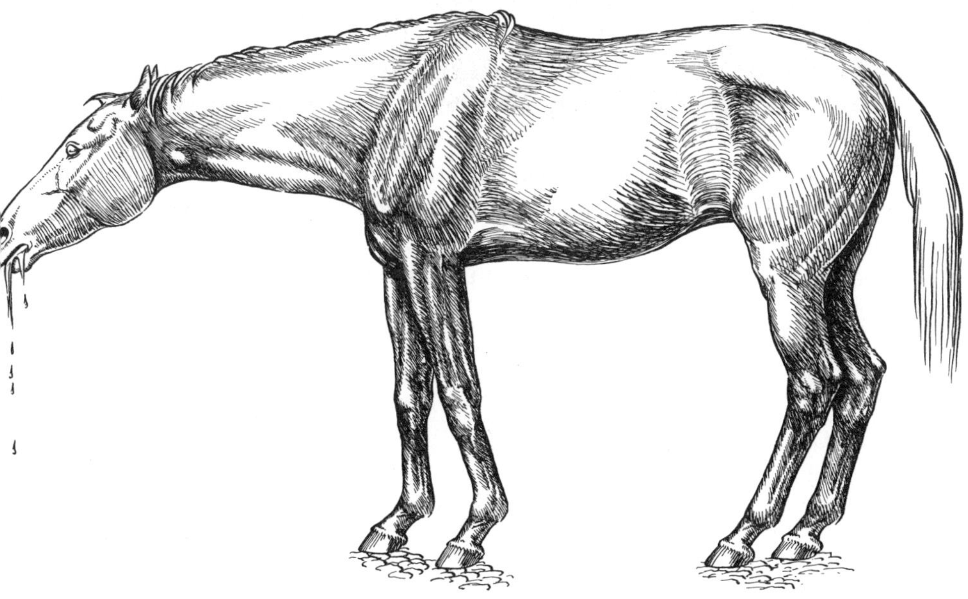

Fig. 43   **A horse with choke.**

or rubber impaction of some lower portion of the intestine may be the result. Baling twine, thrown carelessly about, can be picked up inadvertently and cause either choke or a lower intestinal obstruction. Apples, pears and such can cause choke in the greedy pony or horse who has just broken out and is gobbling up the goodies before being caught.

Choke should be treated by a veterinarian. It may seem simple to cram a broomstick down the pony's throat, but moving the choked material can be a tedious and difficult job. While waiting for the veterinarian, carefully massage the choke mass through the skin (if you can find it in the neck where it usually is). The veterinarian will pass a tube and infuse fluids and push carefully until the mass breaks up and moves on to the stomach. It is most important to get help, instead of hoping that the mass will move on by itself. Usually it stays right there, damages the esophageal wall, and surgery will be necessary to save the horse. That's a mess because the surgery itself is not often successful.

STOMACH

The most serious problem of the stomach, apart from worm infestation, is overfilling with gas and fluid or *acute gastric dilatation*. The horse, unlike most species, cannot vomit. He has no nervous mechanism enabling him to do so. Once materials enter the stomach, then, they can only exit, normally, through the duodenum (the first part of the small intestine). If, for some reason, ingesta cannot move from the stomach to the duodenum, the stomach will overfill with water and food, fermentation occurs and severe gaseous distension is the inevitable result. The distension causes severe pain. The horse sweats and shows signs of extreme discomfort, looking around at his side, rolling, pawing, and so on. The pulse will be fast and weak and the membranes of the eye muddy and discolored. Without prompt, adequate treatment, the distension will cause rupture of the stomach along its greater curvature. When rupture does occur, there will be either sudden shock and death (falling off his feet) or an immediate, but temporary, relief of pain. One may think the animal is recovering, but fatal peritonitis is, of course, quickly on the way.

There are several causes for such distension. The outlet from the stomach, the duodenum, may be blocked or the stomach muscle partially or completely paralyzed. In the latter case ingesta cannot move into the duodenum, and, as a result, there is a functional block.

What can cause blockage of the duodenum? The least common, but most obvious, cause is frank obstruction of the duodenum by an abscess, stricture or tumor. More commonly there is a functional blockage, but that requires some explanation. We have considered how *S. vulgaris*

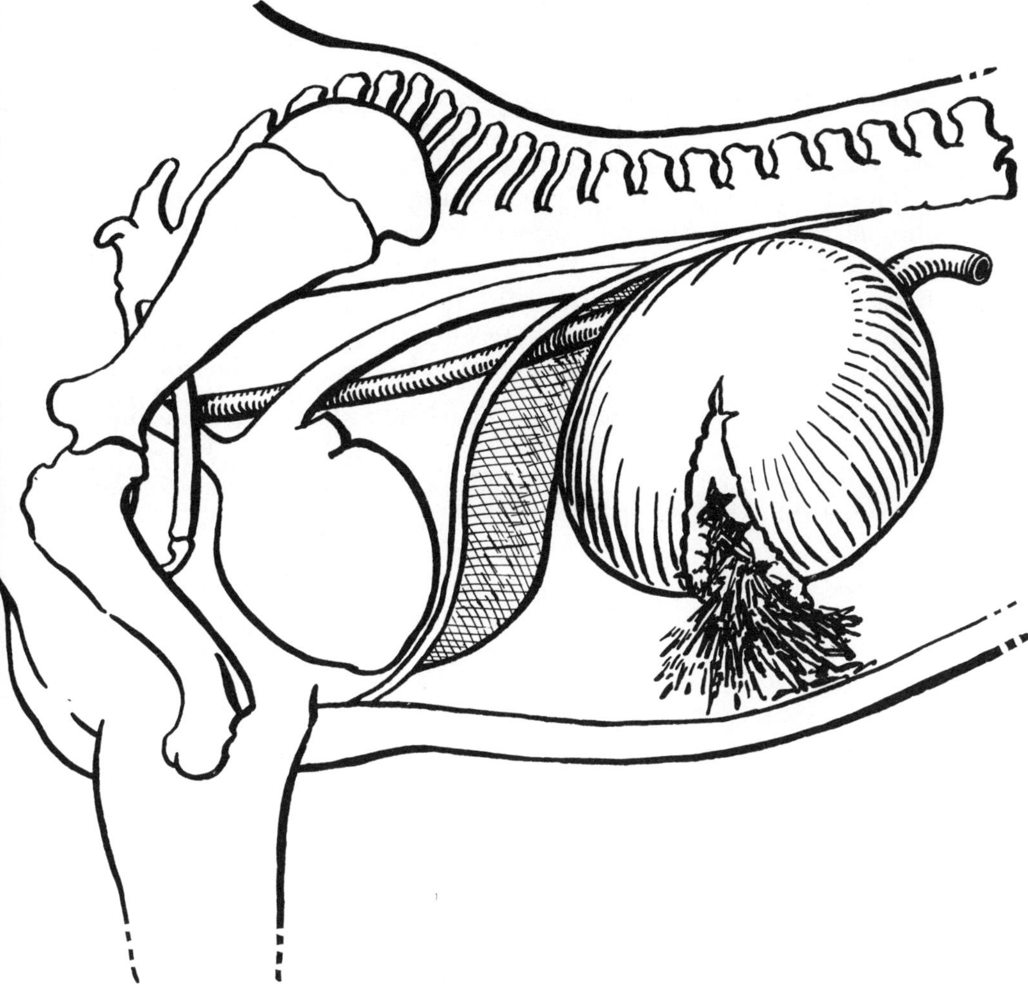

Fig. 44   Rupture of the stomach as the result of acute dilatation of the stomach with food material being dumped into the abdominal cavity.

migrates in blood vessels, obstructing the flow of blood temporarily or permanently. Though preferring the cranial mesenteric artery, the bloodworms can migrate in the celiac artery which supplies blood to the stomach and duodenum (as well as liver, spleen and pancreas). If they do so migrate, the flow of blood can·be reduced, so that the muscle of the duodenum does not contract with normal rhythm and force. If the duodenum does not move normally, ingesta pushed into it by the stomach simply piles up, and the stomach, eventually, can push it no farther. Also, reduction of blood flow to the stomach itself can weaken the stomach muscle, so that it cannot move ingesta into the duodenum.

Paralysis of the stomach muscle, apart from the blood flow reduction just mentioned, can be a most important cause of acute dilatation. It is certainly true that this can happen if a horse overeats on readily fermentable food materials such as grain. The fermentation of the grain in the stomach produces large quantities of gas and short-chain fatty acids, and it is known that large quantities of these fatty acids can paralyze the stomach muscle. (The quantities normally produced in the cecum and colon do not paralyze muscle.)

Any one of the factors mentioned may be operating in any given case of acute gastric dilatation, or several factors may be combining to cause the problem. For example, a feeding of grain which could normally be tolerated may remain in the stomach too long and ferment if the muscle of the stomach and/or duodenum has been slightly weakened by the reduced flow of blood caused by bloodworm larval migration. Neither the grain nor the parasitic damage alone causes the problem, but, added together, acute gastric dilatation is the result.

Given a horse with the acute problem, what does one do? Help should be called immediately. While the veterinarian is on his way, the horse should drink a little water at frequent intervals, if he will. This will wash food passively out of the stomach a little at a time. Do not allow too much water, the stomach problem may be cured only to produce a wicked case of founder (The Lame Horse, pp. 130-134). The veterinarian will pass a stomach tube and try to draw off some of the fermenting material (not easy to do). He will also administer drugs to alleviate the pain and other chemicals to counteract the fermentation of food materials in the stomach. This regimen will save some horses, but, often, the problem is too far advanced too quickly, and medical treatment cannot save the horse. Surgery might be attempted, but it is ticklish at best and probably too late. As usual, prevention is best.

SMALL INTESTINE

Parasitic damage, direct and indirect, is the most important single problem of the small intestine. Complete blockage of the blood vessels to the intestine causes infarction and death from shock and peritonitis. This is the direct damage. Indirect damage is the result of partial blockage of vessels which leads to the several types of malpositions of the small intestine. These are:

1) *Volvulus.* This is a twisting of, usually, the entire small intestine around its attachment (the mesentery) to the upper part of the abdomen. Strongyle

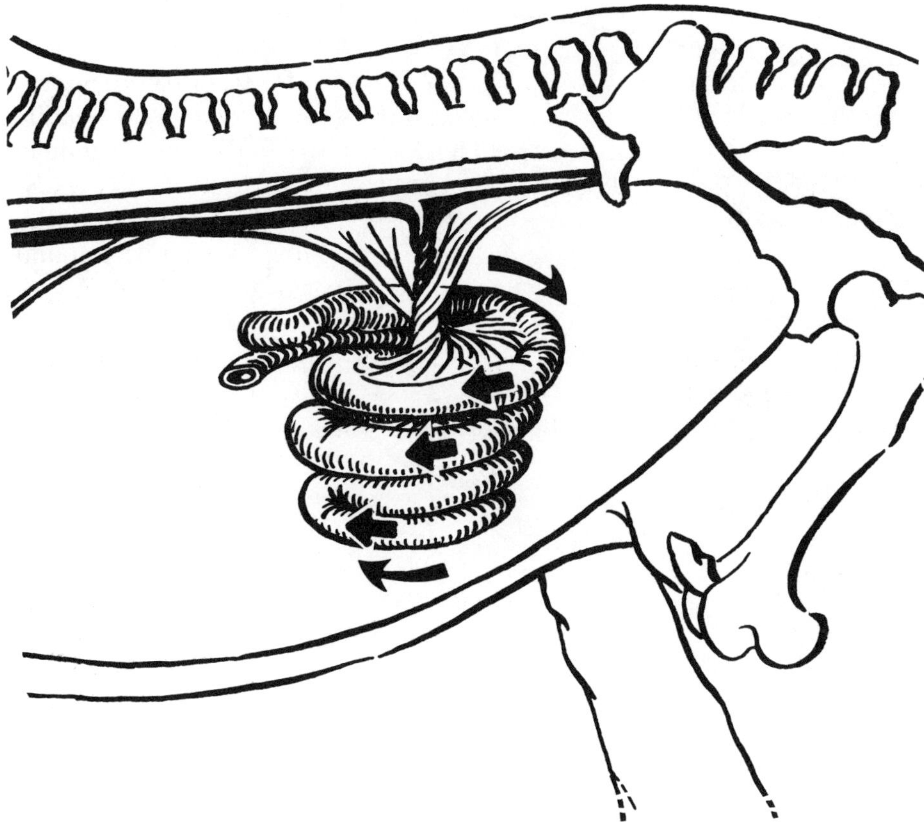

Fig. 45   Volvulus of the small intestine. The gut is tightly twisted on the mesentery as an axis, shutting off the blood supply and killing the gut.

larvae damage vessels supplying the lower end of the small intestine, and the muscle contractions of the gut weaken and slow (this is known as *ileus*). A peristaltic wave moves down the normal intestine, reaches this area of ileus, and overruns it. Since the intestine is fixed at one point, the mesentery, the moving segment tends to turn around the nonmoving segment, and a spiraling twist of the intestine around the mesentery occurs. Once the twisting has occurred, the veins which carry blood away from the intestine are shut down while the arteries continue to pump blood into the wall of the gut. (The walls of the veins are thinner and more easily shut down than those of the arteries.) The gut becomes black red with excess blood, dies, and the animal dies in shock. Only surgery can help and not too often even then.

It has been said that such twists are the result of the horse rolling on the ground. In order to twist the gut in this fashion the horse would have to spin around on his back like a top. Volvulus is caused by bloodworm larvae.

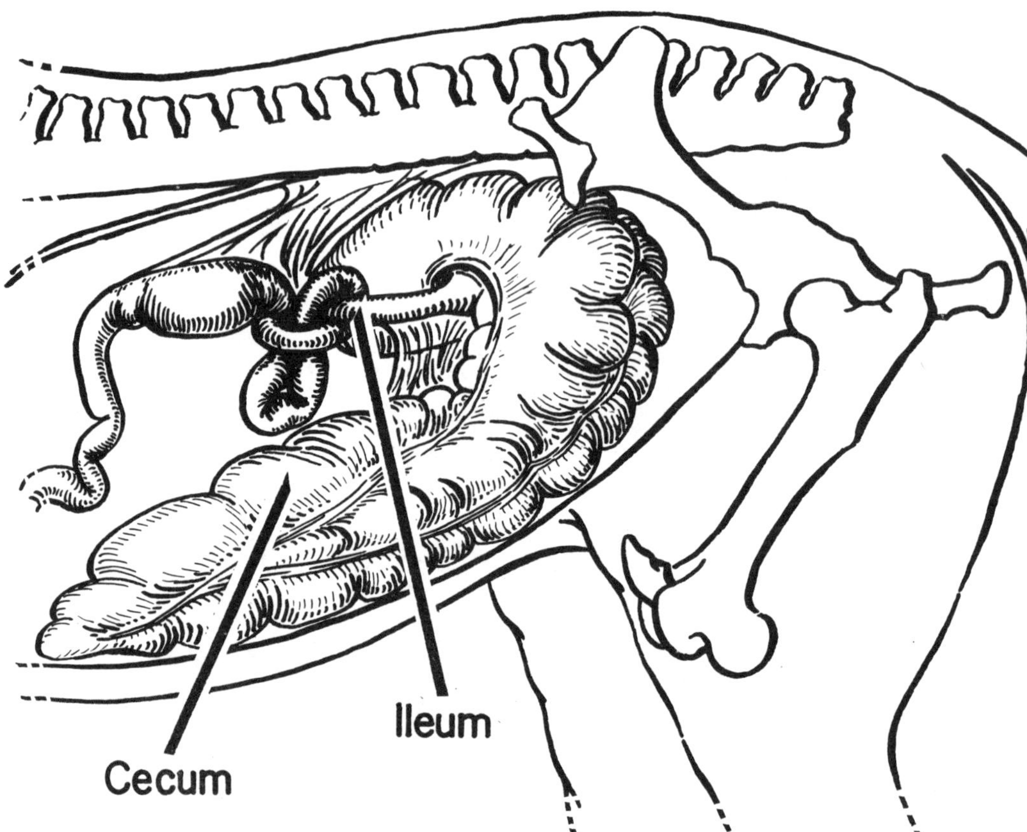

Fig. 46 Strangulation of the small intestine, specifically the last part, the ileum, tying a knot upon itself.

2) *Strangulation.* In this instance the gut ties a knot on itself. The cause is the same as volvulus, a segment of normal gut overrunning a segment which is not moving because of bloodworm damage.

3) *Incarceration.* This is essentially the same as strangulation except that the moving segment of gut breaks through the mesentery as it hits the nonmoving segment and becomes entrapped in the hole thus produced. There are special forms of this incarceration; for example, scrotal hernia discussed earlier, and entrapment of a loop of small intestine through the epiploic foramen, a natural opening between the duodenum and the liver.

4) *Intussusception.* The small intestine may telescope upon itself. This may occur in any part of the small intestine of the foal, but in older horses, mainly yearlings, the ileum telescopes into the cecum. There is a clever surgical technique for this, but, if the horse is wormed regularly and properly, there is no need for it.

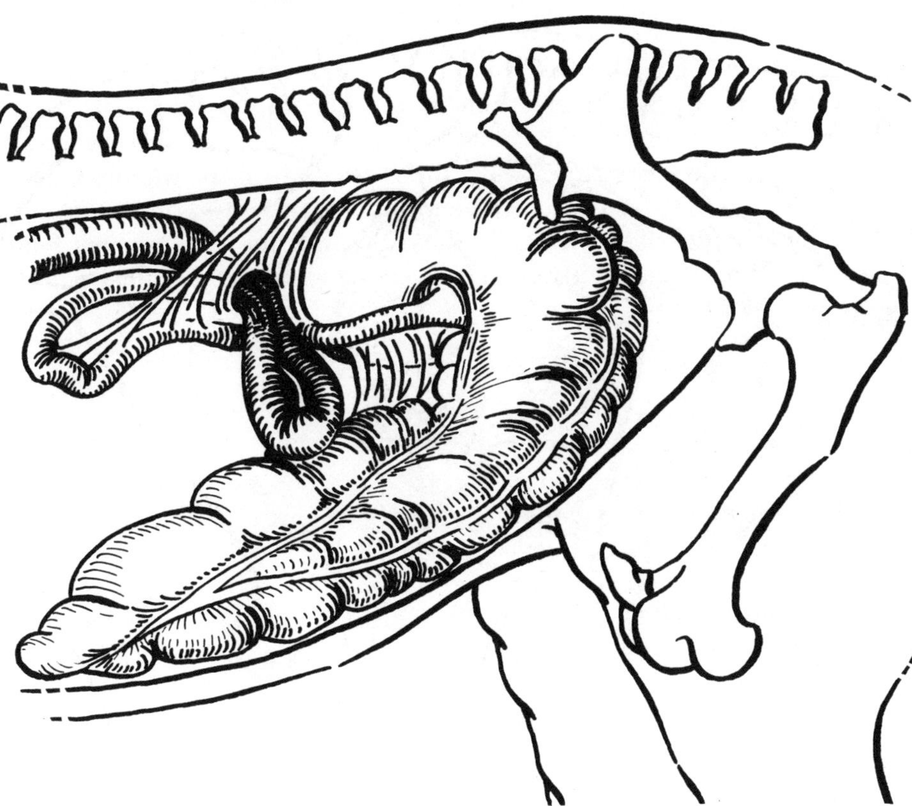

Fig. 47 Incarceration of the small intestine (ileum) through a hole in the supporting mesentery.

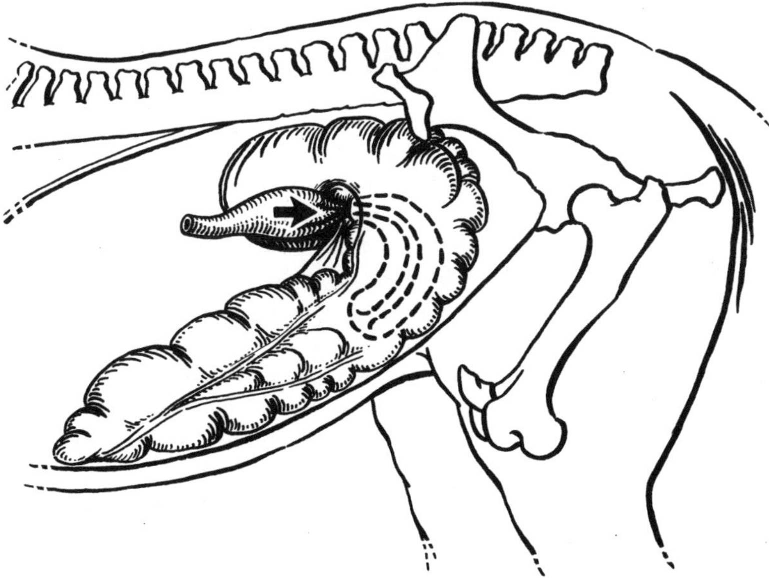

Fig. 48 Intussusception of the ileum into the cecum as indicated by the arrow.

There are other, somewhat less common, malpositions such as rotation of the colon on itself. They kill the horse and the way to avoid them is to worm. One form of strangulation of the intestine occurs with some frequency in older horses and, believe it or not, is not caused by worms! As horses age the fat in their abdomens tends to form tumors called *lipomas* (lip refers to fat and oma means tumor). These tumors may string out on long pedicles and tie half-hitches around the gut, causing fatal strangulation of the gut. Surgery has saved a few animals so afflicted, but age is against the horse.

LARGE INTESTINE

The major problems (need I say it?) are caused by bloodworms. Direct parasitic damage to the colon has already been considered. A condition caused indirectly by bloodworms is of particular importance. While the small intestine can be involved, more often it is the large one. The typical clinical history is that the animal has a single or recurring bouts of not too severe colic. Each time the animal is treated and seems to recover uneventfully. Rectal examination by the veterinarian may reveal impacted ingesta in various parts of the large intestine. The medical treatment (oil, cathartics) combined with massage of the masses per rectum is effective in relieving the signs. Simple and easy. But what is happening; why the impaction in the first place? The evidence is becoming clearer that there is ileus of the segment of large intestine where the ingesta is impacted, and that the ileus is the result of temporary or incomplete blockage of blood flow to the area caused by the migration of bloodworms or emboli breaking off from a bloodworm thrombus in the cranial mesenteric artery.

If this ileus is temporary, and the impaction is relieved, the horse may go on with out another attack. Often, however, one such impaction means that you can expect others in the future, sooner or later. The damage to the vessels is not sufficient to cause frank infarction of the gut but is sufficient to permanently (or nearly so) reduce blood flow and, thus, slow gut movement in the involved area. As a result, the muscle of the gut just above the slow segment will undergo what is called work hypertrophy. That is, the muscle will become thicker and heavier, trying to become strong enough to push ingesta past the slow segment. This is quite comparable to the increase in skeletal muscle mass from lifting weights and such. Unfortunately, this work hypertrophy adds to the problem more than it helps (somewhat like becoming "muscle-bound"), and impaction after impaction is to be expected. The end result, sooner or later, is generally a rupture of the gut just above the involved area with fatal peritonitis. The cecum, transverse colon and pelvic flexure of the large intestine are the areas most frequently involved. These are the areas where bloodworms do the most damage because of certain peculiarities of the anatomy of the blood vessels which we cannot get into here.

As already noted, foreign materials such as baling twine and rubber fences can cause impaction quite unrelated to bloodworms. A rather common foreign body type impaction is known as *sand colic* or sand impaction. It is seen in horses living in sandy areas which, inadvertently, ingest excessive amounts of sand with their food. Horses in such areas should not be allowed to graze short pasturage in order to minimize this problem. A startling and fatal condition which has been called dramatically, colitis "X" involves pooling of large quantities of blood in the large intestine. In fact, this disease is simply severe shock, from a variety of causes, which persists for some time before the animal dies. A full discussion is beyond our scope.

NONFATAL COLIC

This condition is familiar to anyone who has or ever has had a horse. I am, fair warning, going to make the point most strongly that most if not all, attacks of nonfatal colic are caused by the activities of strongyles. Nonfatal colic is broken down, according to who is writing or talking, into a variety of categories, including flatulent, spasmodic, gas, tympanitic, and impaction. The clinical signs can all be explained by the varying degrees of malfunction of the gut caused by worms. It is perfectly reasonable that the migration of the worms can slow blood flow to a segment of gut temporarily, causing clinical signs, and then for the flow abnormality to disappear (the larvae move on) with return to normal of both gut segment and horse.

When the flow of blood is interrupted, the intestinal muscle becomes hyperactive, moving more than normal, and spastic or cramping in nature. This leads to clinical signs of spasmodic colic. If blood flow is not quickly restored, the muscle will relax and become flaccid, and the nonmoving segment of gut fills with gas. This is flatulent colic (also called gas, tympanitic). Spasm in one part of the gut may not permit gas to move along the tract normally, the gas accumulating and causing distension and pain. On the other hand, a gas-filled segment may cause cramping and spastic contraction of the muscle just above it. In many and varied ways, then, the bloodworm-induced blood flow disturbances of the gut muscle can lead to all the recognized clinical forms of colic, fatal and nonfatal.

In more obvious and practical terms it has been noted many times that the incidence of nonfatal, not to mention fatal, colic on a given farm will decrease precipitously and dramatically within a month or two of initiation of a regular and thorough worming program. On one farm, as an example, three to four young horses died every year as a direct result of strongyle infestation with infarction of the large intestine. The veterinarian who did the work for that farm regularly treated at least one case of nonfatal colic per week. He finally convinced the owners to initiate a regular worming program. For the next five years there were no cases of fatal colic on that farm, and the incidence of nonfatal colic immediately declined to about one per month and, shortly, was down to only three or four cases per year (there were about 200 horses on this farm). That story is true, and there are many more just like it.

11
NERVOUS SYSTEM

The nervous system and its diseases, while ultimately fascinating to the serious student, are in many ways most depressing. Diseases of this system are almost always very serious in nature and can rarely be treated specifically or successfully.

The major subdivisions of the nervous system are the brain, spinal cord, peripheral nerves, and the autonomic nervous system. Most peripheral nerve problems have been dealt with in the *The Lame Horse* and will not be considered further here. The autonomic nervous system is of vital importance, being concerned with the automatic, unconscious control of heart rate, breathing, blood vessel tone, gut movement, and bladder function. It is a fact, however, that this system rarely has anything go wrong with it (that we recognize at any rate!), and we shall not devote much time to it.

The brain is composed of numerous subdivisions, only some of which can be discussed. The cerebrum is that large area in which thought processes, specifically those processes characteristic of the species, originate. The area immediately beneath the cerebrum contains the centers responsible for movement, integration of sensory information coming to the brain, as well as centers for the control of eating, sleeping, and sexual activity. More motor areas are found in the midbrain as well as centers for sight and hearing. The cerebellum is a large gyroscopic center, essential for the maintenance of balance and coordination of body movements. Additional vital centers for the cranial nerves, blood vessel control, breathing, etc. are located in the medulla. The medulla blends into the spinal cord which is the "cable" carrying messages back and forth between the brain and the rest of the body.

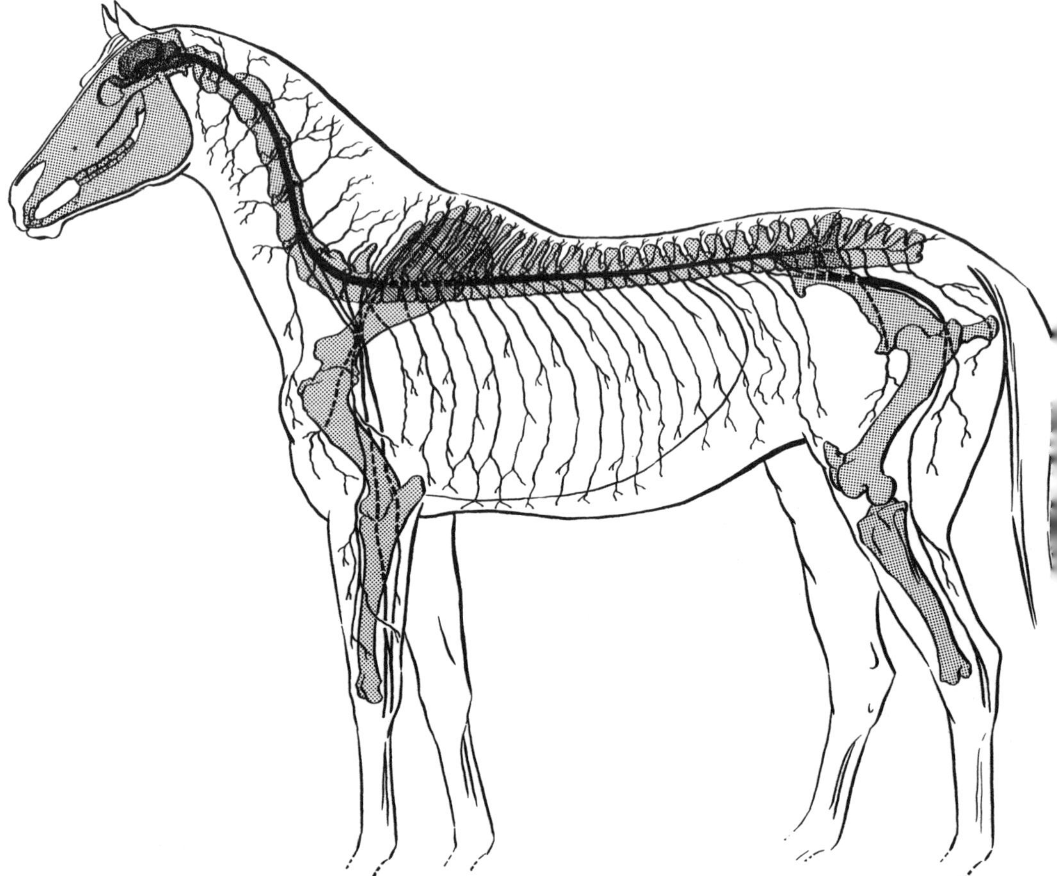

Fig. 49   A general view of *some* of the nervous system of the horse.

ENCEPHALOMYELITIS

Virus diseases which primarily affect the brain will be discussed first. The three most important viruses are known as arbor viruses (ar = arthropod, bor = borne; hence, arthropod or insect carried viruses).

Eastern encephalomyelitis, as the name implies, is most prevalent in the eastern part of the United States but has been found in many other areas as well. The principal carriers of the virus are birds, and the virus is transmitted from them to horses (and humans) by the activities of blood-sucking mosquitos. The mosquito feeds on a bird carrying the virus in its bloodstream. If the mosquito next feeds on a horse or human, it injects saliva after penetrating the skin and can inject the virus along with

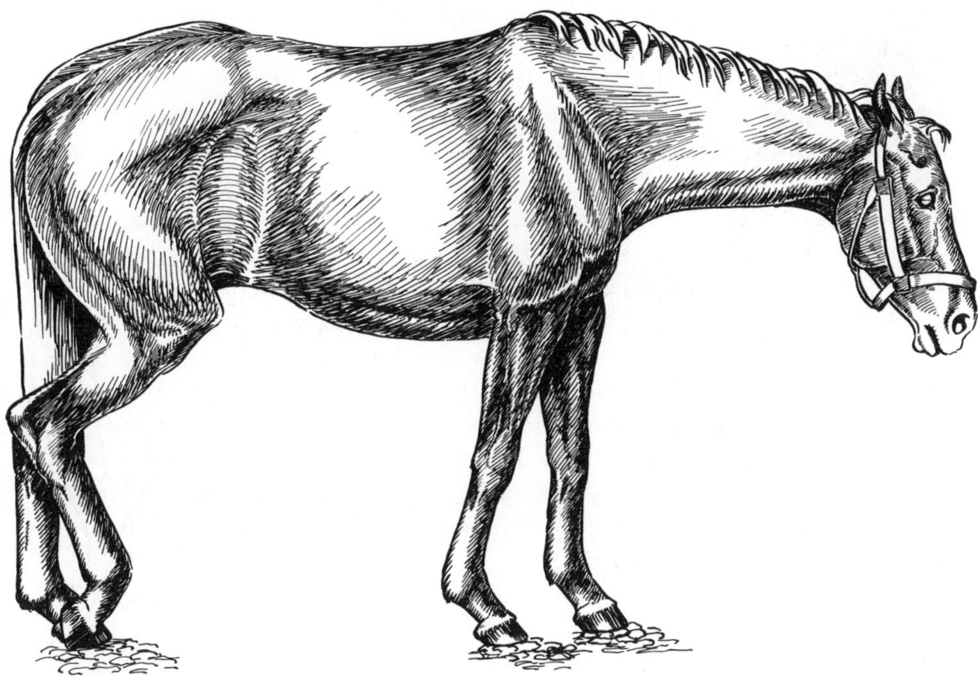

Fig. 50 A horse severely ill with encephalomyelitis. The pattern is that of any severely sick animal.

that saliva. (The saliva is injected, incidentally, in order to prevent the blood from clotting while the mosquito is sucking blood from the animal.) The virus travels in the horse's bloodstream to the brain where it invades neurons (the nerve cells), particularly of the cerebrum, and begins to reproduce itself, using the neuron's metabolic machinery.

The clinical signs may, in the early stages, be those of nervousness and excitability, progressing quickly to delerium, stupor, and severe depression. The animal has a high fever, does not eat, and appears to be unaware of its surroundings. Death usually occurs in a few days. About ninety per cent of the horses that become ill will die.

There is no treatment, but an effective vaccine for prevention of the disease is available. The virus is grown in chicken eggs, killed and formed into a vaccine which is injected into the horse. In high risk areas such as the Atlantic Coastal Plain, the vaccination should be done every year before the mosquito season, and it does provide excellent protection against the disease.

Western encephalomyelitis is a similar disease, most prevalent in the western part of the United States and also transmitted by mosquitos. The clinical signs are essentially identical to the eastern disease, but, on average, less severe. About fifty per cent of affected horses will die. There is an effective vaccine against this agent as well, and, in fact, the two vaccines are combined into one and administered at the same time. It is cheap insurance. One mosquito load of virus is enough to kill a horse.

Venezuelan encephalomyelitis has achieved considerable notoriety in recent years because of the invasion of a virulent strain of the virus into Mexico and Texas. Fortunately, there has been only the one invasion and further evidence of the disease has not appeared in this country. The clinical signs and transmission etc. are similar, in principle, to those of Eastern and Western encephalomyelitis. (There are differences but they are of expert concern.) A live virus vaccine has been used successfully in both humans and horses, and vaccination of all horses in states bordering Mexico has been strongly recommended. The vaccine, since it is live, cannot be combined with others and must be given separately. It is well for you to check with your veterinarian about state laws concerning this vaccination. Recently a killed vaccine has been prepared and combined with the eastern-western vaccine.

There were many claims and counterclaims best forgotten as examples of human fraility as a result of an outbreak of the Venezuelan. One claim, however, was that the vaccine itself could kill horses, and I should like to speak to that important point both about this vaccine as well as others. Vaccines are a great achievement, but they are not panaceas. Not all individuals vaccinated, with whatever vaccine, will respond with an adequate production of antibodies. They may still come down with the disease, in other words, full-blown disease if no antibody has been produced and a milder form if some antibody has been produced. The reasons for such failures or partial failures of vaccination are not completely understood, but the remarks about hypogammaglobulinemia in the chapter on foal diseases are apropos here. Such failures do happen, understood or not, and they must be accepted for now. Secondly, again for reasons which are not completely clear, an individual may respond adversely to vaccination. That is, the individual (animal or human) is allergic to the vaccine and may be seriously harmed by the allergic inflammatory reaction. (This is similar to the damage done to a horse's blood vessels by the allergic reaction to strongyle larvae, as discussed previously.) Unfortunately, this untoward reaction to a number of vaccines (small pox, rabies, Venezuelan encephalomyelitis, for example) affects primarily the brain (postvaccinal encephalopathy is its name) and may kill or permanently maim the animal. That's a most unfortunate thing. There is nothing, however, at the present time that can be done about it. Surely we cannot *not* vaccinate and protect thousands of animals on the chance that we may hurt or kill one. The risk is small, but it is there and must be accepted. Some day, perhaps, as knowledge of disease and its prevention grows, this situation will change, but, for now, we must do the best we can with what we have.

RABIES

Rabies, while one of the most horrible and feared of diseases, happily requires little attention here. Rabies is transmitted by the bite of infected animals, such as dogs, skunks, fox, and bats. Horses are not biting animals (at least they don't often break the skin!), and they are quite adept at taking care of any stray dog or fox that might have ideas about biting them. Cattle are less adept in this regard, and, in some areas at least, are often bitten by rabid fox. One must always have the disease in mind when dealing with central nervous disease in the horse, but it is decidedly rare. While vaccines are available for dog and human, I am not aware that they have been tested in horses.

HERPES VIRUS

The next condition shall be called herpes virus encephalitis with the clear understanding that the role of herpes virus in the disease process is not completely defined at the time I am writing. Rhinopneumonitis virus, coital exanthema virus, and the virus causing cold sores in the human are all examples of the herpes virus group.

A number of limited outbreaks of central nervous system disease have been seen in recent years showing the following clinical signs and course: The animals run a fever and go off feed. They show ataxia (wobbly, unsteady gait) particularly of the rear legs, and temporary, partial paralysis of the tail and urinary bladder (difficult urination). In a few days the fever subsides, and the tail-bladder paralysis disappears. The ataxia becomes less obvious and severe but usually persists in a mild form, reducing the animal's future working usefulness. At postmortem examination scattered, mild lesions are found, particularly in the area just beneath the cerebrum. While the herpes virus has not been definitely isolated during these outbreaks, the pathological changes and some experimental work suggests that virus to be the cause. More research work is needed to answer that question and to provide considerations for prevention. There have been reports of a similar disease problem in some European countries.

FOCAL ENCEPHALITIS-MYELITIS

Another disease which sporadically affects the spinal cord and brain of the horse is called focal encephalitis-myelitis. The cause is not known. It affects individual animals only and has not appeared in outbreaks. Severe destructive inflammatory changes appear in focal areas in the spinal cord and, less commonly, the brain. The clinical signs are quite characteristic, and permanent once they appear. Most animals recover from the acute phase and compensate to some extent for their deficiency but never return completely to normal. There is ataxia of one or more legs, and, without getting into the details, a tendency to drag the foot of the affected leg along the ground when backing or moving sideways.

The cause, as noted, is not known, although some people suspect toxoplasma, a minute protozoan. The disease, while sporadic, is not rare.

MOLDY CORN POISONING

An old-fashioned disease that is still around is moldy corn poisoning. Recent research has indicated that a specific mold is the cause. The mold

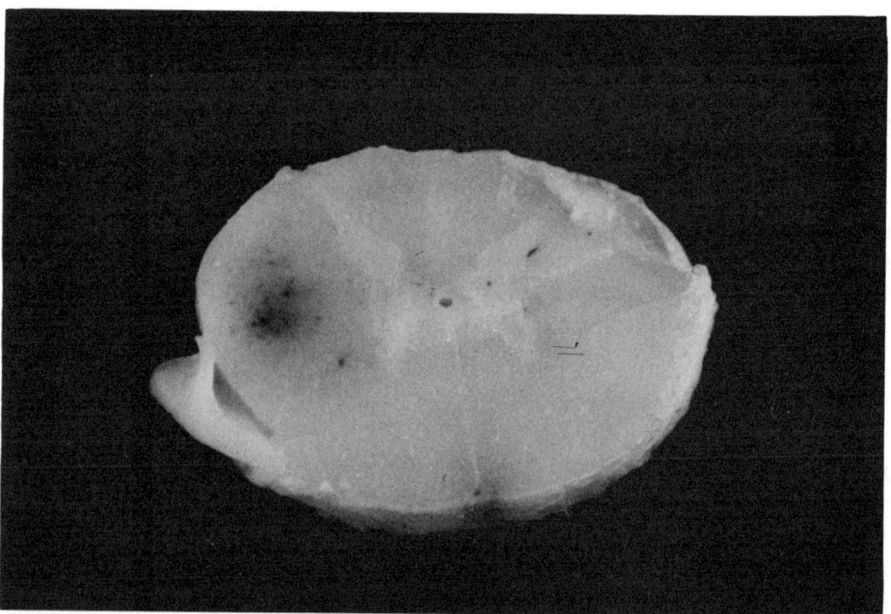

Fig. 51 Cross section of spinal cord with the lesion, dark area, of focal encephalitis-myelitis.

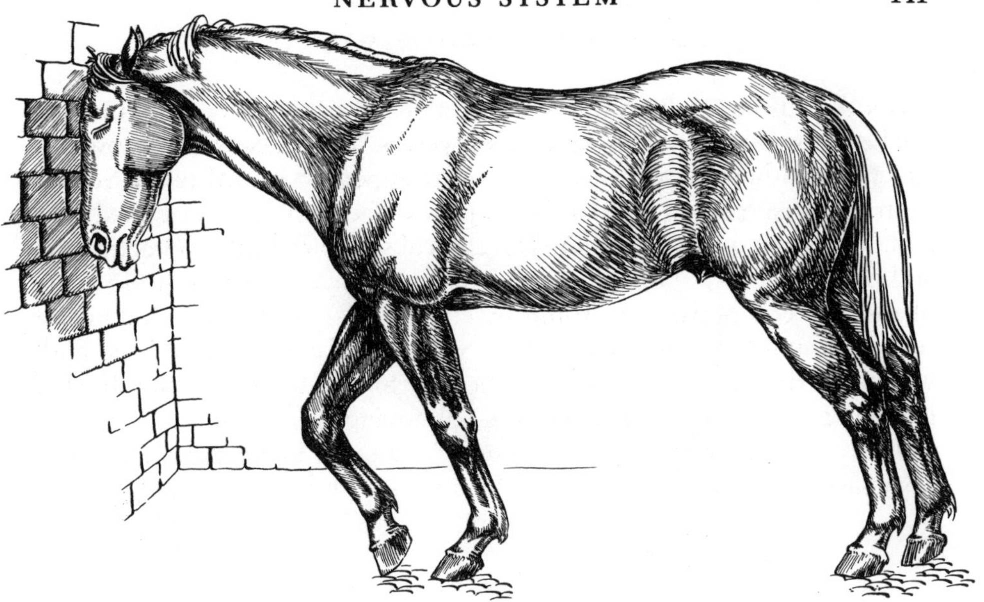

Fig. 52   Dummy, head-pressing horse. This may be seen in the later stages of viral encephalomyelitis as well as moldy corn poisoning.

grows on ears of corn and produces a toxin which, when ingested by the horse, destroys large areas of the cerebrum. Other areas of the brain can be damaged as well, but the worst lesions are in the cerebrum. The clinical signs are similar to those described for all forms of encephalitis. There is no fever, however, and the clinical picture is dominated from the first by stupor and depression. The animal may press its head against the wall for hours at a time, walk through fences, and appear completely blind and unresponsive. The damage is permanent, and the horse usually dies within a week after onset. There is no vaccine or treatment. Avoid moldy corn!

There is another condition, somewhat similar, restricted to the western United States. It is known as nigropallidal encephalomalacia. It is a severe, local destruction of parts of the brain following ingestion of either yellow star thistle or Russian knapweed. Again, the damage is permanent and prevention the only approach.

TETANUS

Tetanus is caused by the toxin produced by the bacterium, *Clostridium tetani*. This organism is ubiquitous in the environment of the horse.

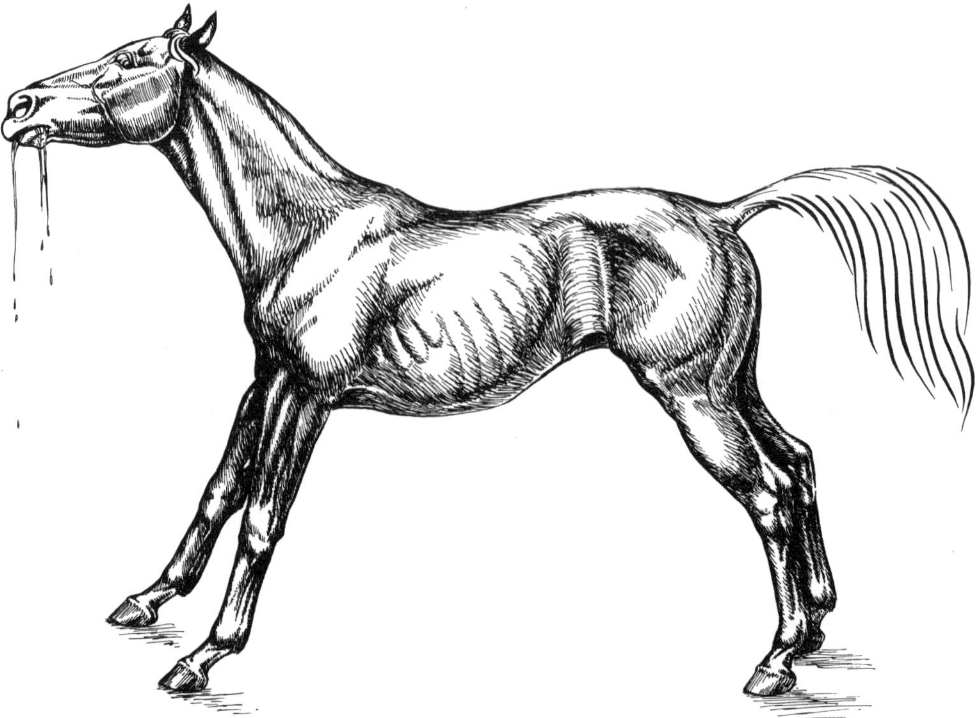

Fig. 53 Tetanus with the typical rigid, sawhorse attitude.

Many horses, in fact, appear to carry the bacteria in their digestive tracts. If the tetanus organism enters a wound, it grows and reproduces, elaborating a potent toxin. This toxin blocks nerve synapses, so that the skeletal muscles either contract sporadically or continuously without control. The horse assumes a sawhorse attitude when the muscles are contracting spastically. In the early stages of the disease, the slightest noise or movement may cause the third eyelid to flash across the eye. Once clinical signs appear, most horses will die a difficult, agonizing death. Treatment is rarely successful and long drawn out. The only answer is routine toxoid administration to all horses with booster doses when necessary.

FORAGE POISONING

This is a subject of great vagueness and difficulty but must be dealt with because it is not at all uncommon. The evidence presently available indicates that most, if not all, cases of so-called forage poisoning are actually the specific disease, *botulism.*

Botulism is caused by the toxin of another clostridial organism, *Clostridium botulinum.* This toxin blocks the transmission of nerve impulses from the nerve ending to the muscle and, as a result, the muscles are paralyzed. The clinical signs usually appear suddenly as generalized weakness, specifically wobbly rear legs and trembling of the triceps muscles just above the elbow. When the horse tries to eat or drink, food and water runs out of the nostrils because of paralysis of the muscle of the throat (pharyngeal paralysis). The animal may die quickly or linger for some time, apparently related to the amount of toxin ingested.

Treatment is usually not effective, but the following may be tried: The veterinarian will attempt to administer oil and fluids by stomach tube in an effort to flush out the intestinal tract. He may administer, by slow intravenous drip over ½ hour, a liter or two of saline containing 5 mg. of neostigmine and 1 ml. of 1-1000 epinephrine. This should be repeated every 8 hours. I prescribe in detail here because many veterinarians are not aware, through no fault of their own, of this formulation. The idea is to allow proper functioning of the nerve endings while the toxin is being broken down and removed from the horse. Some horses will recover with this treatment. Others will not recover but will show at least temporary relief or partial alleviation of symptoms. I consider a positive response good evidence that the problem is botulism, even if the horse does not eventually recover.

When the diagnosis is reasonably certain (and the response to treatment helps in that regard), the horseman must get to work. The premises must be carefully and meticulously combed, looking for the source of the toxin, be it contaminated feed, or a decomposed rat or rabbit in a bale of hay. Botulism organisms grow in dead animal tissue, among other places. Silage is dangerous for horses because the airless (anaerobic) conditions in a silo are ideal for the growth of the organism. Cows can apparently degrade the toxin in their large stomach if there is not too much of it. Horses cannot. Cows, then, can happily eat and grow fat on botulinum-contaminated silage which kills horses.

LIGHTNING STRIKE

Lightning strike is not rare in horses on pasture. If possible, horses should be stabled when a storm is threatening. If not, horses, like cows and humans, will tend to gather under trees to avoid the rain. The bolt of lightning heading for the tree hits the horse, and he is dead—right now. It is, I suppose, possible for a horse to be hit and survive, but I know of no example. Lightning may strike the tree and the horse be knocked down by sheer fright, tree branch or whatever, so that one thinks it has been hit by the bolt and recovered.

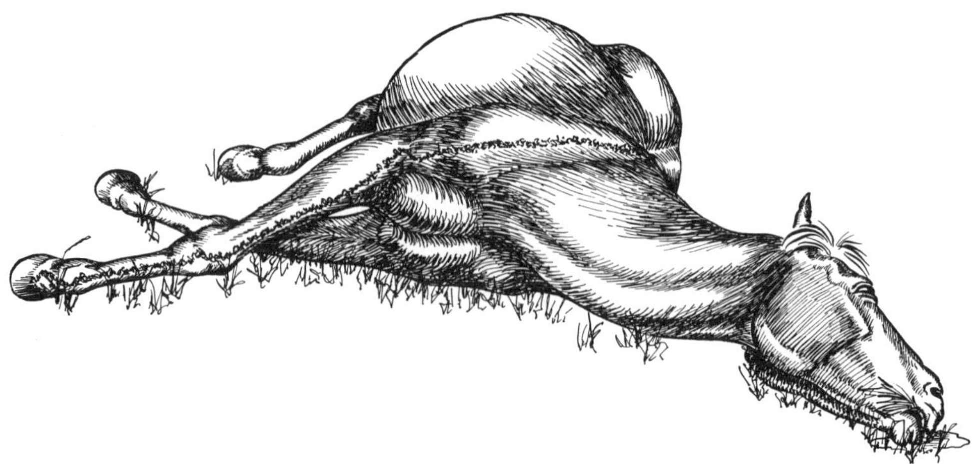

Fig. 54   Horse struck and killed by lightning. Grass in the mouth indicates the sudden death. The characteristic, though not invariable, singeing of hair from withers to hoof is shown.

The major problem is determining that it was, indeed, lightning which struck the horse, and that it did not die of some other, potentially dangerous, disease. More than once horses thought to have died of lightning strike were autopsied and another cause of death found. The postmortem diagnosis can be made with absolute certainty only if there are burn tracks, singeing of hair in an arborizing or linear pattern on the skin. The tracks usually run from the withers down the foreleg to the coronary band. If these tracks are not present, the autopsy will reveal only a greatly enlarged spleen (shock spleen) and congestion of most body organs. The diagnosis, then, can only be made by elimination of other causes and the history of a storm. Occasionally, the electrical charge may cause such powerful tetanic contractions of the muscles of the struck horse that the back is broken at about the 12th thoracic vertebrae. When present, this fracture is further evidence for lightning strike.

TRAUMA

Trauma is a common cause of brain damage in light horses. A foal's head may be fractured, the front of the head between the eyes, by the kick of a mare, usually because the foal forgets which udder belongs to him. In older horses skull fractures occur most commonly when the animal rears up and strikes an overhead obstacle: door frame, stable overhang. The horse may simply rear up and fall over backward, causing the same type of

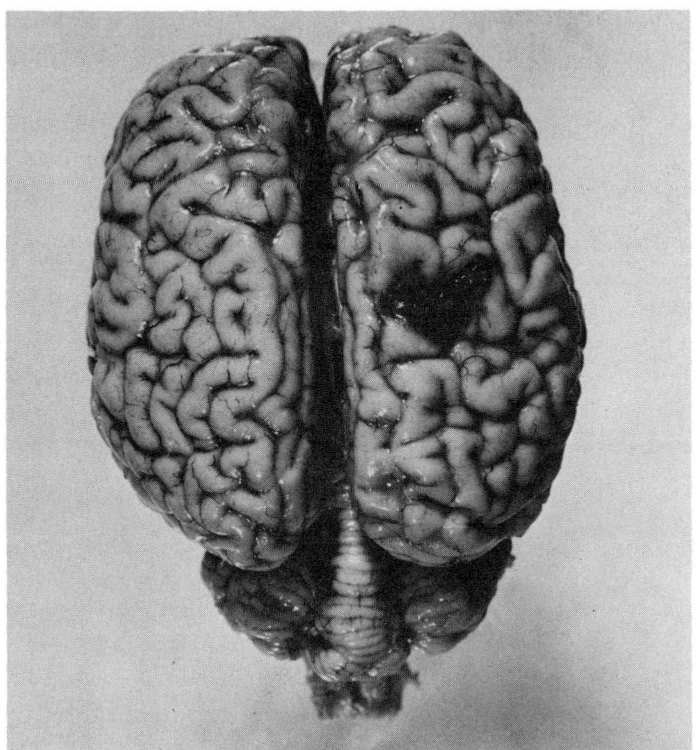

Fig. 55   Top view of brain of a foal. The dark area is damage to the brain done by the kick of a mare. The skull was fractured and the brain damaged.

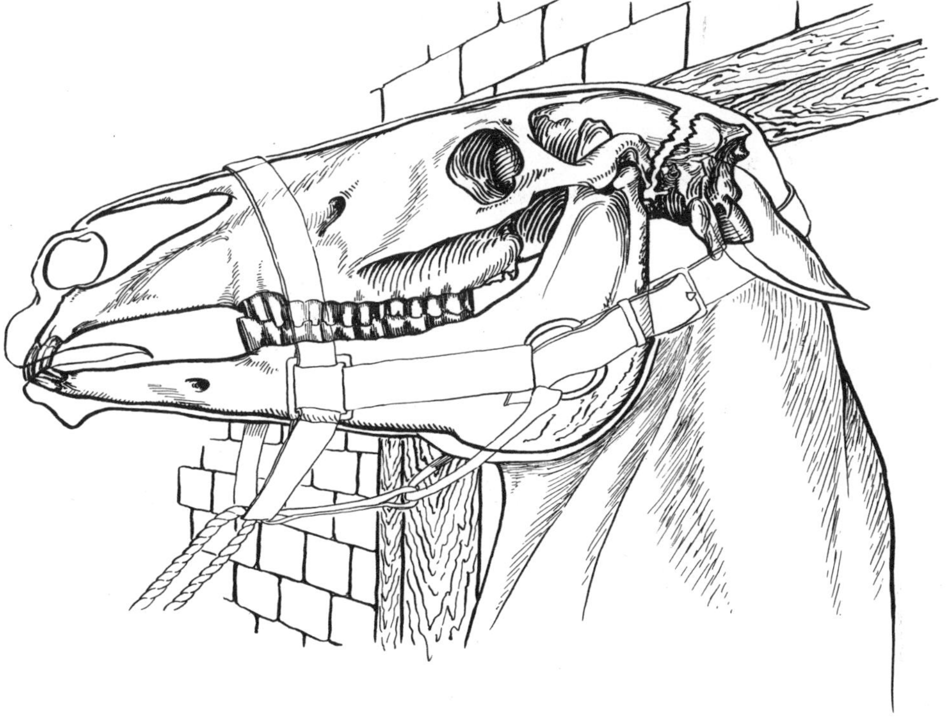

Fig. 56   Horse rearing up, striking head on overhead object and fracturing the skull along the jagged lines. This is a most serious injury.

fracture. The poll strikes the obstacle or the ground and levers the back part of the skull away from the rest of the skull. After the event the animal is unconscious for a period. When consciousness returns the animal cannot get up. It may be difficult, even with x-rays, to determine that a fracture has occurred since the bones break along natural attachment lines, and there may be little separation between the broken edges. The fracture almost invariably breaks through certain bones of the ear, however, and blood will be present in one or both ear canals. If not obviously running from the ear, a cotton swab may be run into the ear to determine if blood is present. In my experience blood in the ear is *prima facie* evidence of skull fracture. Although the affected horse may not die, the massive bleeding in and around the brain has done permanent damage, and the animal will have to be destroyed, sooner or later.

If a horse strikes his head as described, goes down, and gets up on its own within a few hours, the prognosis is somewhat better. The animal may survive for a long time, but one must be aware of the possibility of permanent, residual neurological defects. In particular, damage may have been done to the rear part of the brain (occipital lobe), and the

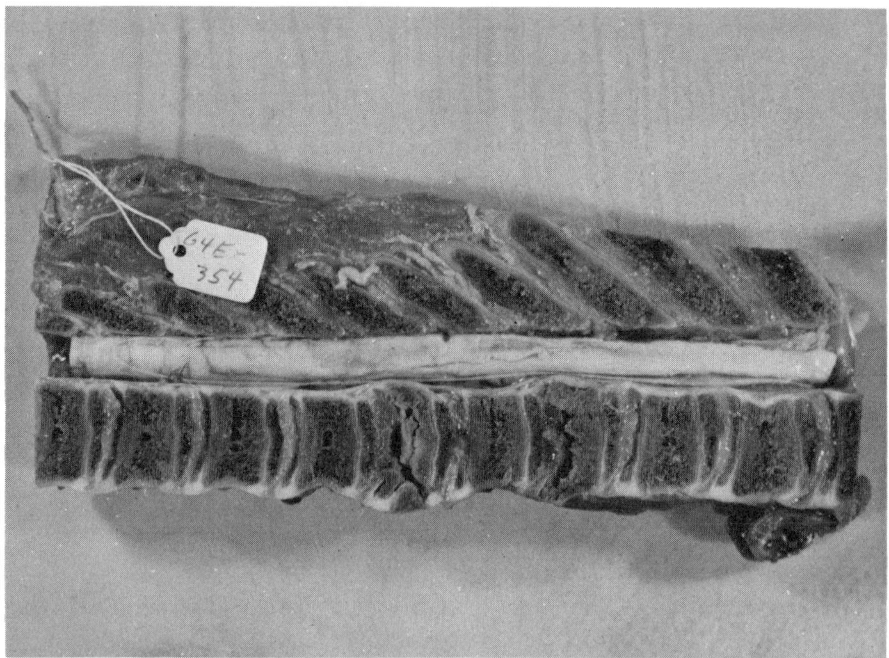

Fig. 57 Two fractures of the backbone of a foal that tried to leap a "too-high" fence. The bulging of the fractured vertebrae against the white spinal cord may be seen.

animal may be completely or partially blind because this is the area of the cerebrum involved with conscious sight.

Horses can also break their own backs (see Tetanus). Foals trying to jump fences which are too high can do this. The animal will be down and unable to rise, though conscious. The veterinarian can determine that fracture has probably occurred, and that the animal should be put down.

Foals and older horses may somersault over a fence or other obstacle and tear apart the vertebrae in their necks. If down and unable to rise after such an accident, the prognosis is hopeless. If the animal gets up, it may hold the head and neck very rigid and be unwilling to move the neck even to eat. Damage has obviously been done, but most such animals will, in time, recover completely. Water and feed must be placed so that the horse can reach it without bending his neck.

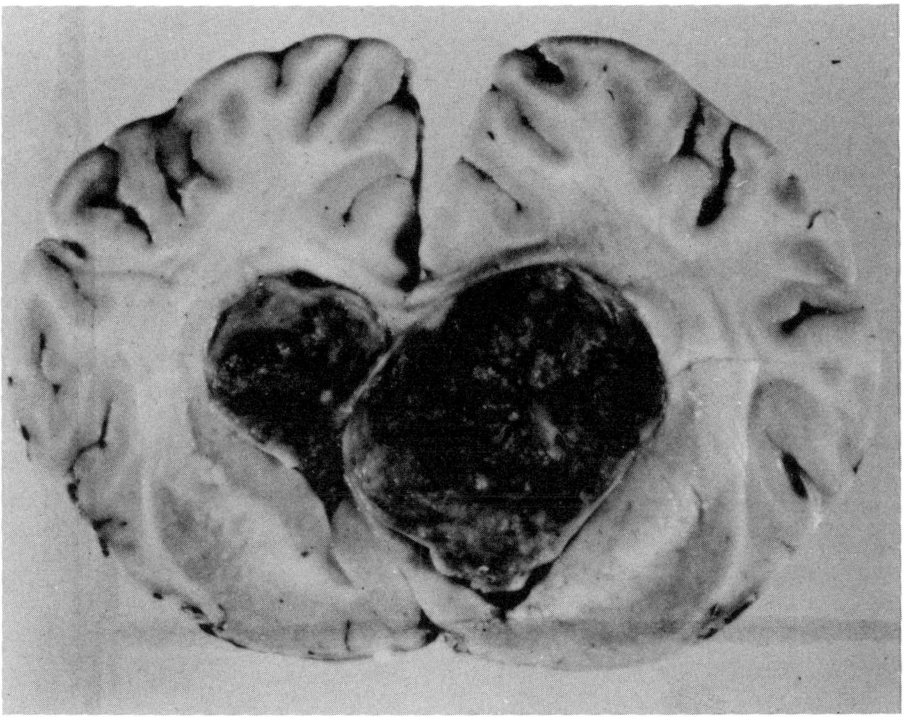

Fig. 58   Cross section of brain of a horse with a cholesteatoma, the darker, mottled areas in the center, which causes distinct neurological signs. It is not common.

OTHER NEUROLOGICAL CONDITIONS

Tumors and abscesses of the brain or spinal cord in the horse are extremely rare. Melanomas may invade the spinal cord. Tumor-like masses, cholesteatomas, occasionally develop within the brain. The animal circles to one side only, and there is a personality change from tractable to nasty. There is, of course, nothing to do about any of these problems. Neurosurgery in horses is not yet!

Certain other important neurological disorders: wobbler, neuritis of the cauda equina, radial paralysis, etc. have been discussed in detail in The Lame Horse to which the reader is lovingly referred.

12
BLOOD

In this chapter some disorders of the blood shall be considered as well as some other problems at least marginally related to blood. Some conditions, specifically neonatal hemolytic disease, have already been considered.

The condition of the blood completely dominates the thinking of some horsemen. They seem to believe that if only the blood could be made good enough and rich enough, that damn horse would win! Most of the time this is wishful thinking, and it is something other than the blood which is not right. There are two common "states" of the blood in the working horse which require consideration.

HEMOCONCENTRATION

Hemoconcentration is, basically, too many red blood cells for the amount of fluid in the bloodstream. The horseman may think this a fine thing because the hemoglobin and red blood cell counts are so high. In fact, it often means that the horse is chronically dehydrated, not receiving enough water to replace that lost during training and / or racing. All horses should have water continuously before them. This chronic dehydration may form part of the condition to be discussed next.

NONSPECIFIC TRAINING ANEMIA

Anemia, a decrease in the numbers of red blood cells and the amount of hemoglobin, can occur in horses kept in training for protracted periods and, therefore, shut up in stalls for protracted periods. The precise nature of this anemia is not known, but one may suggest that prolonged training and work without let up may simply exhaust the animal, his blood-forming system as well as everything else. The best of stall-feeding regimens may well not be completely adequate, and low-grade nutritional deficiency can develop. Shots and pills and magic potions through needles are not the answers. Fresh air, green grass and rest are the answers.

PIROPLASMOSIS

This in an infectious disease which specifically affects the red blood cells. It is caused by a minute protozoan of either of two species, *Babesia caballi* and *Babesia equi*. They are transported by ticks which infect the horse by injecting the protozoa at the time they bite the horse to suck blood. The disease occurs primarily in subtropical areas and has been reported in the United States only in Florida.

The clinical signs are fever (not invariably, however), depression, inappetance, edema of the legs and lower part of the abdomen and eyelids. Hemorrhages may be seen on the third eyelid. Other signs such as jaundice, weakness, colicky signs and a weak, thready pulse may be present. Anemia is the major sign. It is caused by the breakdown of the red blood cells because of invasion of those cells by the protozoan. The horse may die or recover to become a symptom-free carrier. The protozoa are present in the blood of the carrier horse and capable of being transmitted to another horse by ticks or needles. The horse is immune as long as it is a carrier. In the United States, the carrier state is eliminated by treatment, while in countries where the disease is widespread no treatment is used.

The acutely ill horse can be treated with specific drugs and supportive therapy. If initiated early, the treatment is often successful.

EQUINE INFECTIOUS ANEMIA

This is an old scourge of the horse that is still with us and probably long will be with us. The recent development of a serological test (the Coggin's test) provides a means for detection of the disease not previously available. EIA is said to be a virus disease peculiar to the horse. It is transmitted from horse to horse by biting insects or contaminated needles and instruments. Under farm conditions, the horseflies are said to be the important vectors.

Once infected the horse may show signs of acute, subacute or chronic disease. In the acute form the signs are very similar to those described for acute piroplasmosis. The subacute disease is a prolongation or continuation of the acute stage. The animal may seem to be recovering from the acute attack only to have recurring attacks of varying duration and severity interspersed with periods of normalcy.

The chronic case seems to have recovered completely but may show occasional, variably severe periods of illness. These recurrences occur during periods of work or stress. These symptom-free, chronic horses are said to serve as a source of virus, through needle or horsefly transmission, to other horses.

Control programs are now in progress in many states using the Coggin's test as the basis for detecting infected horses. The reader is advised to check with his state veterinarian's office for the relevant laws before buying, selling or shipping horses.

As so frequently happens control programs are set in motion before full information and, indeed, full thought has been given to the disease problem. There are many aspects of the cause and natural history of this disease which are far from clear at present. Considerably more research of a high order of sophistication needs to be done before practical control programs can be developed. For example, if the horsefly is, indeed, the major vector, it would seem that research to develop strategies for controlling it should be of first priority. I should rather kill a lot of them than a few horses!

LEPTOSPIROSIS

This disease has been reported in horses infrequently. It is caused by one or another spirochaetal organism. The disease can be a significant problem in man, dogs, cows and pigs. In the horse, however, it is, at best, a subclinical problem. Horses certainly are exposed to the disease and react by producing antibodies. Significant clinical disease in the horse, however, is very rare. The relationship of leptosirosis to moon blindness has been long and hotly debated, and there is no more evidence now than ever that there is a real relationship. The evidence, indeed, points more strongly to onchocerca microfilaria as the important causative agents.

LEUKEMIA

This is an all too familiar malignant disease. Virtually all species can be afflicted, and the horse is no exception. The lymphoid cells of the body grow wildly and without restraint and eventually kill the animal. A virus or viruses seem to be the cause as the evidence is accumulating.

The clinical signs are rarely clear-cut and can appear in animals of any age. There is gradual wasting and debilitation and specific signs depending upon which organ the malignant cells are filling at any given moment. In a young horse, for example, the malignant cells often accumulate in the ileum of the small intestine, and the clinical signs are those of intestinal obstruction.

There is nothing to be done. The treatment strategies applied to the human have not been developed for horses.

SPLEEN AND LYMPH NODES

The spleen is a singular and interesting organ. It serves as a storehouse for red blood cells with the capability of storing those cells until they are

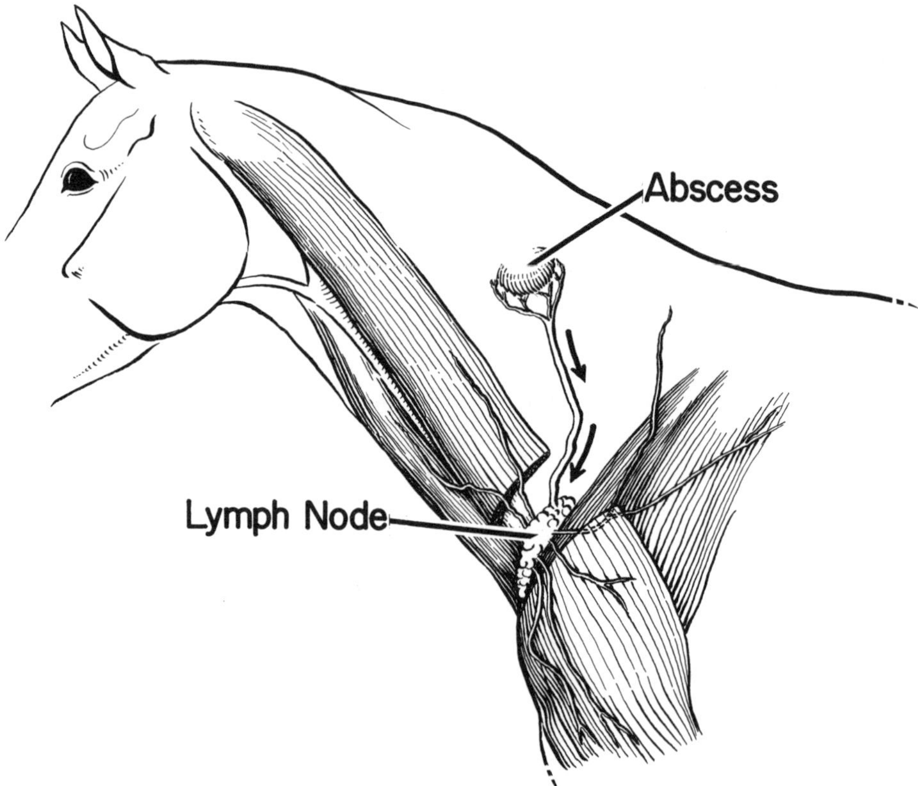

Fig. 59   Representation of one of the functions of lymph nodes. An abscess in the neck "drains" by way of lymphatic vessels to a regional lymph node. The lymph node serves as a defense against further spread of the infection.

called for by exercise, stress, etc. The spleen also serves as a major area for the production of antibodies and for the removal of foreign material and microbes from the bloodstream.

This "cleansing" function of the spleen which it shares with the liver, lymph nodes and bone marrow deserves further comment. In the organs mentioned there are macrophage cells which constitute the reticuloendothelial system. These cells are strategically located along the routes of blood flow in order to remove foreign materials, worn out and dead cells, etc. The macrophages engulf (eat, since macrophage means "big eater") these materials and digest them, so that they no longer contaminate the blood stream.

Lymph nodes are important sites, as is the spleen, for the production of antibody, as well as providing a home for the macrophages. Lymph nodes are strategically located to provide a second line of defense against infectious processes. If an abscess forms on the neck, for example, bacteria in the abscess may escape and travel in the lymphatic vessels, looking, one might say, for a new place to live. The lymph vessels pass through regional lymph nodes, however, and the bacteria are trapped and destroyed by the macrophages (and a few neutrophile friends). The lymph node may be damaged, but it has done its job of stopping the spread of the infection.

13
SKIN

Skin disorders in horses are near legion and cause considerable concern because of their visibility. It is said of the human dermatologist that he has the perfect medical practice because his patients never get well and they never die. There is some truth in that for the horse and some of his skin problems as well.

RINGWORM

Ringworm usually appears in groups of horses, particularly young animals. Discrete rounded or irregular patches of scaly dermatitis with loss of hair are scattered over the body. The patches tend to enlarge in a roughly circular manner. There are a number of different fungi which cause this lesion, and they can be differentiated by laboratory study of skin scrapings. Most of these infections are self-limiting, running their course in seven to eight weeks. Stable equipment and tack should be carefully and scrupulously cleaned and kept that way since the disease is readily spread from horse to horse. The veterinarian can recommend appropriate treatment.

ALOPECIA

Alopecia or loss of hair is, in fact, a general sign of something wrong with the skin and not a specific disease. Either temporary or permanent hair loss may accompany ringworm. A horse with severe, systemic disease may lose much or all of its hair but, with recovery, the hair will grow back. The normal shedding of the winter hair coat may, in an occasional horse, be uneven and progress to frank alopecia. Usually the hair grows back in a reasonable time.

CONTACT DERMATITIS

This is an important cause of focal hair loss accompanied by oozing and weeping of the skin. The diagnosis may be immediately suspected because of the relationship of the skin damage to girths, bridles, blankets, etc. A common form is the loss of hair over the rearquarters of a foal with diarrhea (known as "scalding"). Chemical agents used in the manufacture of tack items as well as fly sprays, sheep dips, etc. can all cause dermatitis. Any such chemicals used around or on horses should be diluted and handled *precisely* as described by the manufacturer or the veterinarian. Pigeons and chickens roosting over horses can and will deposit droppings which cause contact dermatitis along the back. Filthy, urine-soaked stalls are another cause, this time, along the belly and on the legs. The obvious treatment, of course, is to remove the offending material. Local application of salves and ointments to protect the areas from further damage by rubbing and biting is indicated.

PHOTOSENSITIZATION

In this condition, unpigmented areas of skin will become reddened, swollen, and itch when the animal is exposed to sunlight (ultraviolet rays). The chemical substance causing this problem can be derived from several sources and circulates in the bloodstream. When exposed to ultraviolet light, the chemical absorbs the rays and gives off energy which kills nearby cells, setting off an inflammatory reaction. Pigmented skin prevents the rays penetrating to the chemical in the tissues just beneath the skin.

The source of the chemicals may be plants, particularly Saint John's wort. More commonly photosensitization in horses is associated with chronic liver disease. A pigment normally formed from chlorophyll in the intestine (phylloerythrin) is absorbed into the bloodstream and excreted by the liver through the bile ducts into the gut. If the liver is damaged (cirrhosis), the phylloerythrin may not be completely excreted by the bile route and, therefore, will circulate to the skin and act as a photosensitizing agent.

ALBINISM

While true, complete albinism may not occur in horses, there are animals with an incomplete form. The color of the skin is due to cells containing melanin pigment in the skin. If the pigment is not there, the skin is white, and such skin is obviously prone to sunburn and photosensitization. The melanin pigment absorbs the sun's rays and prevents liberation of large amounts of energy in the skin. Clearly blond humans sunburn more readily than blacks, and the same is true of light horses as compared to bays and blacks.

SUMMER ECZEMA

This is a highly pruritic (itchy) inflammation of the skin which is probably an allergic reaction to flying insects as already discussed. While steroid ointments will help alleviate the itching, prevention is the real answer.

LUMPS AND BUMPS

Of these there are many. We have already mentioned the lumps caused by habronema larvae. *Sarcoid* is a benign fibrous tumor which can appear anywhere on the horse's body and is particularly common in young animals. Some disappear on their own, but they are easily removed surgically.

Certain fungi, particularly *blastomyces*, can cause granulomas (lumps) in the skin. *Mastocytosis* is an uncommon, probably true tumor that can be removed surgically. *Leukemia* occasionally involves the skin. *Carcinomas*, slowly malignant tumors, may appear anywhere on the body but seem to be most frequent around the sheath, particularly of older geldings.

Melanoma occurs, as is well-known, in older grey horses (most of the time). They appear as dark lumps on the undersurface of the tail and around the anus and vulvar area. They can spread to internal organs and kill the horse. They should not be interfered with surgically. There is some evidence that spread is more active and vigorous after surgical "stirring up."

LYMPHANGITIS

While not specifically a skin disease, lymphangitis comes close enough

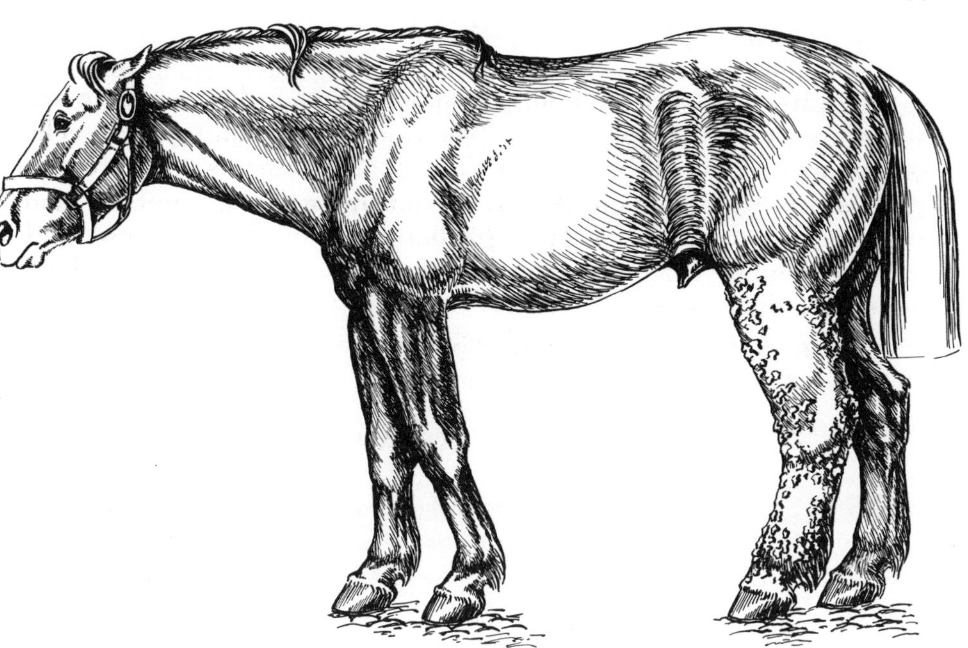

Fig. 60   Horse afflicted with lymphangitis. The rearleg is thickened and the skin scurfy.

to be considered here. The lymphatic vessels beneath the skin are infected and filled with pus. The surrounding tissues become swollen and inflammed, leading to an overall, enlarged, painful "milk leg." This almost always affects one or both of the rear legs. There are two defined causes and several others which are still not clear. The first known cause, a fungus, *Histoplasma farciminosum*, has not with certainty been found in this country. That is fortunate because the condition spreads rapidly from horse to horse and is very difficult to treat.

The second cause, also a fungus, is *Sporotrichium schenkii*. It, too, is difficult to treat but griseofulvin is effective.

The more common, garden-variety cases of lymphangitis are probably caused by the bacterium *Corynebacterium pseudotuberculosis* or some other species of corynebacterium. Secondary infection with streptococcus is common. It is important to decide, early in the course of the disease, the precise cause. A biopsy should be taken for histological and cultural study. If the exact cause is not determined, the wrong treatment can be used, and the lesions become so far advanced and scarred that the leg or legs are permanently deformed. Antibiotics for long periods is the treatment of choice for bacterial lymphangitis while griseofulvin has been shown to be effective for sporotrichosis.

C. pseudotuberculosis, at least in some of the western parts of the United States, can cause severe abscesses in the chest region and, less often, on the inside of the rearleg or along the ventral body wall. Flies may transmit the infection. Surgical drainage and antibiotics are used in treatment.

AURAL PLAQUES

Whitish, slightly elevated, crusty plaques may occur inside the ears. There aural (ear) plaques may persist for long periods. The cause is not

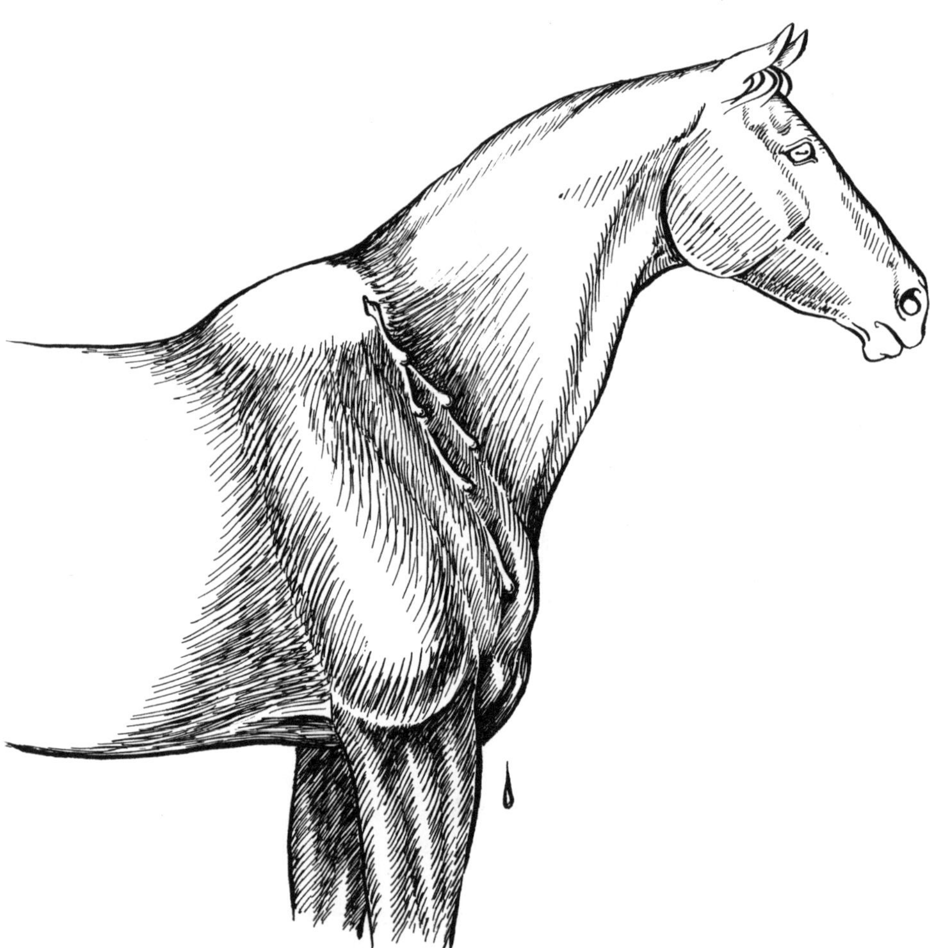

Fig. 61   Fistulous withers. The swelling over the withers has burst and pus is running down over the front of the shoulder.

known, and there is no effective treatment. Black flies feeding on the
plaques may cause considerable irritation.

FISTULOUS WITHERS AND POLL EVIL

These conditions are not seen with any frequency in modern times but

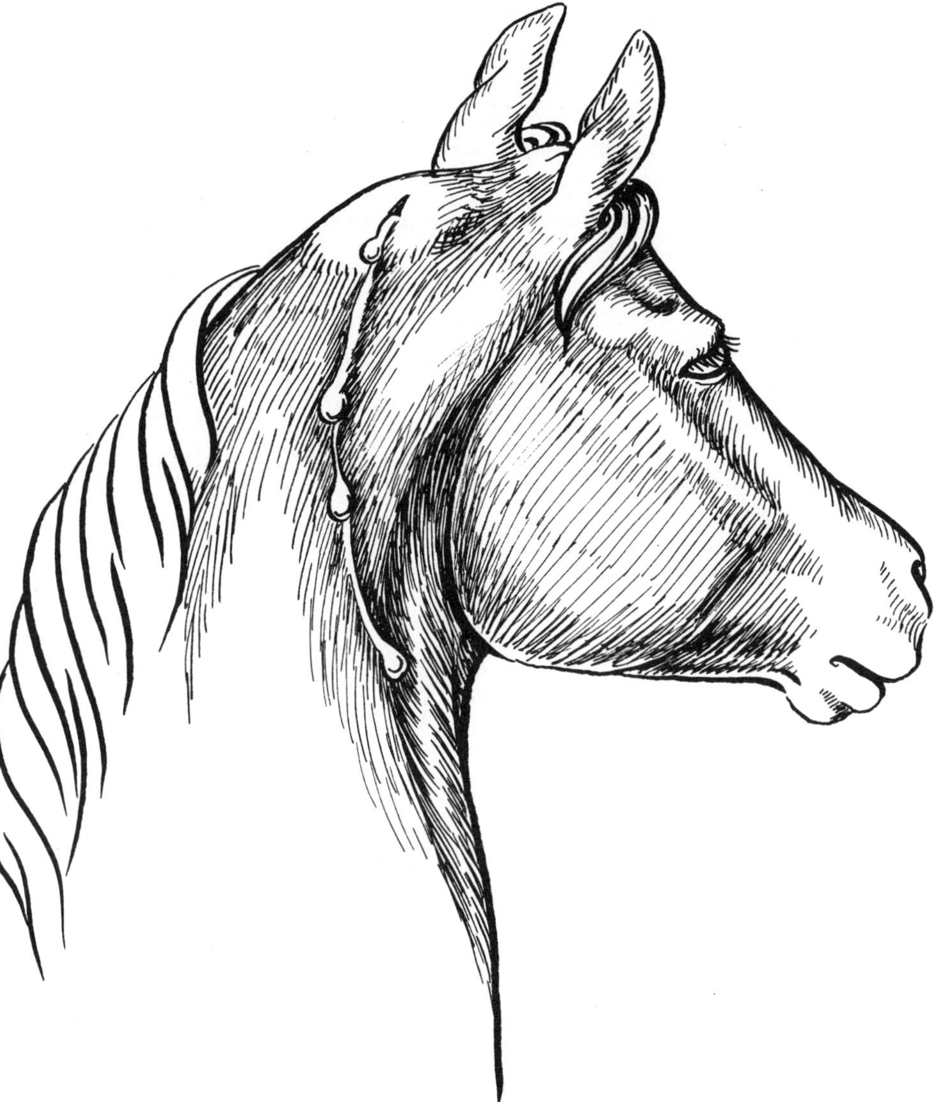

Fig. 62   Poll evil. The swollen, inflammed bursa just behind the ears has burst and
is draining.

were both common and important in the draft horse days. We'll have more to say about that below.

Fistulous withers is an infection which begins in a bursa normally located on top of the spines of vertebrae at the withers. Initially there is a soft, painful swelling in the area, and the horse resents and actively resists the seating of collar or saddle. The abscess, for thus it is, may dissect down into the tissues of the neck and/or break open and drain. Neither surgical incision nor antibiotics are completely satisfactory once the disease process is well-established. Probably a combination of surgery and antibiotics in early cases is the best strategy.

Poll-evil is an entirely comparable process occurring in a bursa located just behind the poll on the top of the horse's neck. Treatment is the same, and just as messy and difficult, as fistulous withers.

Both of these infections apparently result from rubbing of harness on the affected areas, abrading the skin and allowing two bacteria to invade the bursae. These two bacteria, actinomyces and brucella, acting in concert, cause the abscess. They are primarily pathogens of cattle, and it is true that these conditions were and are more common in horses that live together with cattle. Brucella has been largely controlled or eradicated in cattle in the United States and that, together with the decline in draft horses and the fact that most light horses are not kept with cattle, has reduced the incidence of these diseases to an occasional rarity.

14
HEAD

TEETH

There are several things which can go wrong with the teeth. The so-called wolf teeth may have to be removed because they erupt crookedly (but more often are removed because it is traditional to do so). In older horses the premolar and molar teeth may wear too much, producing sharp edges which can cut the cheeks. This can be taken care of by floating (rasping) off the sharp edges. While of merit in the older horses a great deal more of this floating is done in young horses than is really necessary.

The *fourth upper cheek tooth* may become diseased and have to be removed. This tooth is prone to genetic defects in the formation of its surface which allow food materials to enter the tooth. Inflammation and necrosis occurs. The condition is probably similar to caries in the human. A defective tooth of this sort has to be removed (we don't fill them!), and that can involve rather extensive surgical procedures. The roots of the horse's teeth are quite long, and the tooth cannot be readily pulled out. Horse teeth wear down slowly with age, and the roots become shorter and shorter as the teeth move out in response to the wear. In sandy areas the teeth may wear much more rapidly than usual.

As is well-known the age of a horse can be determined to a certain extent by examination of the teeth. The time of eruption of the teeth and the progress of wearing provide clues to age. Many light horses, however, do not obey the rules. One can see two year old mouths in five year olds and vice versa. Age determination by the teeth, then, is an aid and not absolute fact.

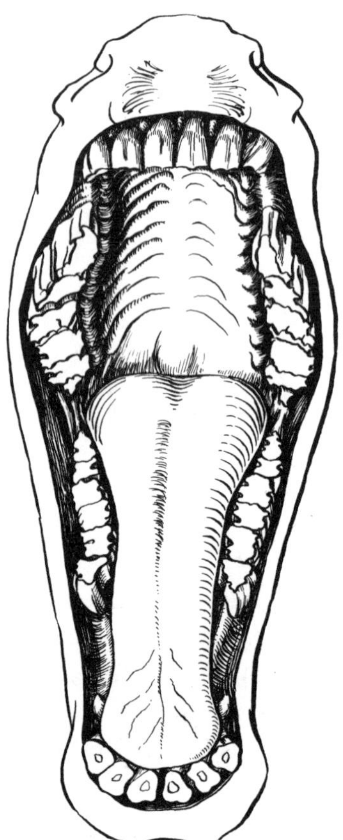

Fig. 63   An exaggerated view of the horse's mouth showing the incisor, premolar and molar teeth.

A foal may be born with (although it may not become obvious until later) a localized swelling of, most commonly, the lower jaw. This is a bony-walled, cystic structure known as an *odontogenic cyst*. It has other names as well, but that one is bad enough. This is a congenital defect of tooth formation leading to tumor formation. When small these lesions can be removed surgically with some hope of nonrecurrence. Once they have attained some size, which they do very rapidly, they are difficult or impossible to deal with, and the animal has to be put down.

SINUSES

The horse, as other species, has a series of sinuses or air spaces located in the skull and communicating with the nasal passages. Neither in man

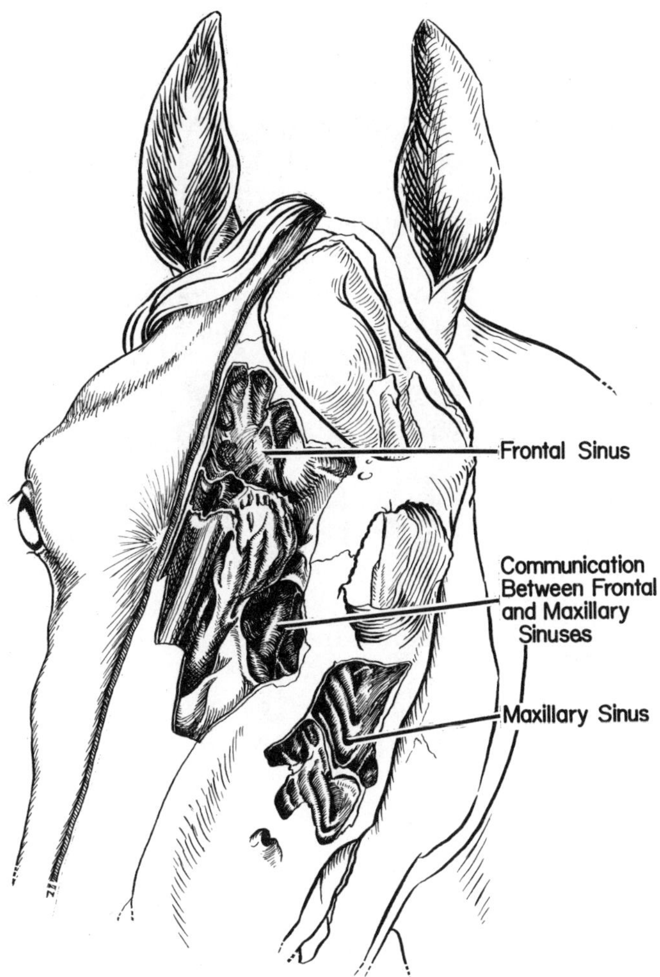

Fig. 64 Some of the sinuses of the horse's skull.

nor animals is the exact function of these spaces known. In any case, infection of the sinuses can occur, often associated with that diseased fourth cheek tooth we talked about. Tumors (carcinomas) may also begin in a sinus. The clinical signs will be a one-sided, stinking nasal discharge and perhaps (with the tumors) swelling of one side of the face. Prompt diagnosis is essential. If the problem is a tumor, the prognosis is essentially hopeless. Infections, on the other hand, can usually be treated and, if an infected tooth is the cause, its removal will be necessary.

EYE

The eye is obviously of great importance, and I have little to say about it. The reason is simply that the eye is nothing for anyone but the professional to deal with. Just a little bit of home-doctoring, and the eye will be irreparably damaged. Even a veterinarian may wish to refer eye problems to a specialist. Inflammation in or near the eye may only be dust or fly irritation, but there may be something such as an ulcer present and, if by delay or home remedies, that ulcer is not promptly taken care of, it can perforate, and the whole eye collapse and be lost.

There is always a little fringe of black nodules hanging from the upper edge of the iris. These are called *granula iridies* and are normal. Some horses have irregular pigmentation of the iris (wall-eye). It, too, is normal.

Ecessive *tearing* should always be checked. It may be the result of simple eye irritation or a blocked tear duct. Tears produced by the lacrimal gland wash continually over the eye and drain into the nose through the tear duct. The opening of the duct into the nose can become plugged, but is readily opened by the veterinarian.

The third eyelid is a protective shield and "window washer" for the eye. A slow-growing carcinoma may develop on the third eyelid (inflammed eye, excessive tearing!). It can be removed, in the early stages, with good results.

MOON BLINDNESS

This condition is also known as periodic ophthalmia or recurrent uveitis. It is the commonest severe eye disease of the horse. Either one or both eyes may be affected. There is pain, reddening, excessive tearing, and reluctance to open the eyelids. The attack may subside in some days only to recur at varying intervals until the eye is completely opaque or destroyed. The recurrent nature of the attacks led to the old idea that the phases of the moon had something to do with the disease.

The cause or causes are still in dispute. Riboflavin deficiency, leptospirosis, and onchocerciasis all have their adherents. I bet on the last. Treatment is mainly designed to alleviate the clinical signs. Corticosteroids should be particularly beneficial both locally and by systemic injection.

VICES

Some few vices of horses have already been discussed here and there

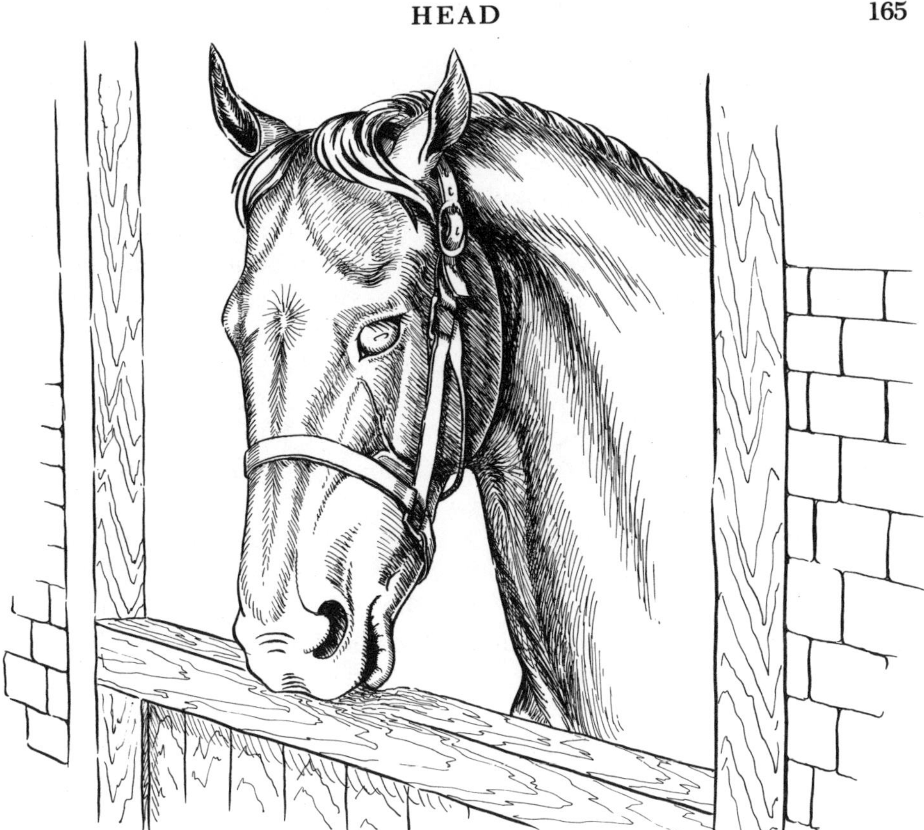

Fig. 65   A cribbing horse.

through the book. One or two more may be mentioned. *Cribbing, weaving* and *stall-walking* are all vices, if that's the proper word, which develop in stabled horses. The cribber grasps a firm object with its teeth and grunts, apparently swallowing air. A variation of cribbing is the animal which constantly chews the wood in its stall. The weaver simply stands in the stall and sways, hour after hour. The stall-walker is obvious.

All of these habits apparently develop because of the boredom and isolation of a naturally gregarious animal. These habits rarely appear in herd groups at pasture. Once established the habits are very difficult or impossible to break even if the animal is turned out with others of its own kind.

Prolonged stabling is simply not natural for the horse and, if it must be resorted to for whatever reasons, such annoying habits must be expected and lived with.

15
MISCELLANY

Inevitably there are some conditions not considered in previous chapters which should be mentioned.

TURNING-OUT SYNDROME

This is a strange entity sometimes seen in horses which have been in heavy training and racing and are suddenly turned out to pasture for a rest or because of lameness. The syndrome is characterized by general weakness, quick tiring with any degree of exertion, depression, loss of weight, dehydration, depressed levels of blood sugar, anemia, and diarrhea. The horse may die or gradually return to normal after a prolonged period. It has been suggested that this is caused by Addison's disease; that is, improper functioning of the adrenal glands and subsequent inadequate levels of steroid hormones. While complete proof is lacking that the adrenals are involved, it is said that rest and hormone therapy will return a number of these animals to normal. I have no personal experience to go on.

HEAT STROKE—EXHAUSTION

These are significant problems of the horse. In the case of exhaustion the horseman's desire to compete (for example in a trail ride) may exceed the training and ability of his mount. If endurance riding is your thing, consult an experienced rider and your veterinarian about a training program long before you plan to compete. You and the horse will be spared much grief! It is true that some horses can be pushed so far that they become exhausted enough to go into shock and die.

Heat stroke occurs more frequently than one would think. Heavy work and training in hot, humid weather can precipitate an attack. The horse becomes depressed, staggery, and sweating stops. The rectal temperature can be amazingly high. Immediate treatment with cold water, preferably running constantly from a hose, is necessary. The veterinarian can help with intravenous fluids which will help to wash hemoglobin (released by heat breakdown of red blood cells) through the kidneys. There have been stallions suffering from heat stroke from running the fences on nonbreeding days (mares in heat being led by their paddocks) who have died a week later from hemoglobin blockage of their kidneys.

NUTRITION

For many years we have been feeding horses or allowing them to feed themselves without knowing at all what and why we were doing in scientific terms. Despite this ignorance, the results have been remarkably good. I have hectored at some length about nutrition in *The Lame Horse* and will spare you more. Research is going on now at several centers, and everyone is looking forward to the results. While inadequate nutrition can cause problems in horses, one should not fall into the trap of blaming nutrition without justification. The problem is really worms!

THE END

Despite all that has been said there are diseases and "states of ill-health" that cannot be diagnosed or understood no matter how hard we try. The horse goes off feed, runs a slight fever, and is somewhat depressed. Rest, tempting food, clean and abundant water, sun, green grass and all is soon right again. What happened? We may not know, and, say like the physician, "I don't know, but it's going around."

INDEX